AF710197

When Your Child Hurts

CENTRAL UNITED METHODIST
CHILDREN'S LIBRARY

Charlotte Adelsperger

AUGSBURG Publishing House • Minneapolis

WHEN YOUR CHILD HURTS

Copyright © 1985 Augsburg Publishing House

All rights reserved. Except for brief quotations in critical articles or reviews, no part of this book may be reproduced in any manner without prior written permission from the publisher. Write to: Permissions, Augsburg Publishing House, 426 S. Fifth St., Box 1209, Minneapolis MN 55440.

Scripture quotations unless otherwise noted are from the Holy Bible: New International Version. Copyright 1978 by the New York International Bible Society. Used by permission of Zondervan Bible Publishers.

Photos: Dave Anderson, 13; Fred Gonnerman, 27; Camerique, 43; Wallowitch, 57; Jean-Claude Lejuene, 61, 97; Larry J. Kopp, 79; John Keskinen, 87.

Library of Congress Cataloging in Publication Data

Adelsperger, Charlotte.
WHEN YOUR CHILD HURTS.

1. Parents—Prayer-books and devotions—English.
2. Children—Diseases. I. Title.
BV4529.A32 1985 242'.4 81-68639
ISBN 0-8066-2161-3

Manufactured in the U.S.A. APH 10-7088

1 2 3 4 5 6 7 8 9 0 1 2 3 4 5 6 7 8 9

For Ron and Alberta Heil,
who are an inspiration to me
and
in loving memory of their son
Mark, who, abiding in Christ Jesus,
demonstrated that courage is contagious.

"Fear not, for I am with you,
be not dismayed, for I am your God;
I will strengthen you, I will help you,
I will uphold you with my victorious right hand."
—Isa. 41:10 RSV

Contents

Perspective

Despair and grief
flash across
the delicate screen
of our lives.
Agony—
no easy answers.

In time, we encounter
a Comforting Light
projecting through
it all.
Peace—
still, no easy answers.
Our response:
walk on and on
in that Light.

Preface

A mother tells of holding her feverish daughter on her lap, her own arms shaking.

"Oh, mommy, keep holding me," the little girl cried.

"As I wrapped my arms more tightly around her," the mother relates, "I wondered who was going to hold *me* through all the crises of her condition."

How parents like this one seek to be upheld and empowered lies at the center of this book. It was written especially for the parents of children who are receiving extensive medical care because of an illness, an accident or a chronic physical condition. It comes as a friend to keep those dads and moms from feeling so alone.

A sizable number of parents with children needing medical care have contributed out of their souls to the contents of these conversational prayers and interviews. As one parent pointed out, "We all start at a different place, and all our situations are unique." Although every situation could not possibly be covered, you will find certain prayers coinciding with what you are going through. Each is based on someone's true experience.

I have focused on the needs of parents who want to be strengthened in order to care more effectively for their hurting children. In most of the interviews, names have been changed to protect family privacy.

The dedication in the front of the book will help you to understand what inspired me to begin this project—witnessing the vital faith of my twin sister, Alberta, and her husband, Ron, during their son's seven-year battle with leukemia. The way in which 13-year-old Mark Heil lived the Christian adventure has touched my life deeply. In his last exhausting fight for life, only a few hours before he went to heaven, he declared, "Something good has got to come out of this." Mark's words remain with me, and I pray that this book will be part of that something good. For you see, I shall never forget Mark nor all the precious parents, including his own, who have talked so openly with me.

Collecting material for *When Your Child Hurts* has been a moving experience. I have marveled at parents' willingness to give of themselves, even while they were hurting, in order to help other parents. As one chaplain put it, "In living through a child's illness, it makes a world of difference if parents can understand and accept their feelings, especially when they pray."

May what you read here help you get in touch with your own feelings, and prompt your own spontaneous prayers and reading of the Scriptures. It will make a world of difference! God bless you as you turn to him for your specific needs.

Charlotte Rist Adelsperger
Prairie Village, Kansas

Part One

Fear Not, for I Am with You

Upheld

I know not how God moves,
but that God comes quickly,
into our struggles
into our pain
into our deepest joys—
if invited.

His immeasurable love
and mystery
masters our striving,
smiles on our progress,
enables our victory.

When all seems as losing,
God through Christ
upholds his children
in puzzling power,
lifting us even
over death.

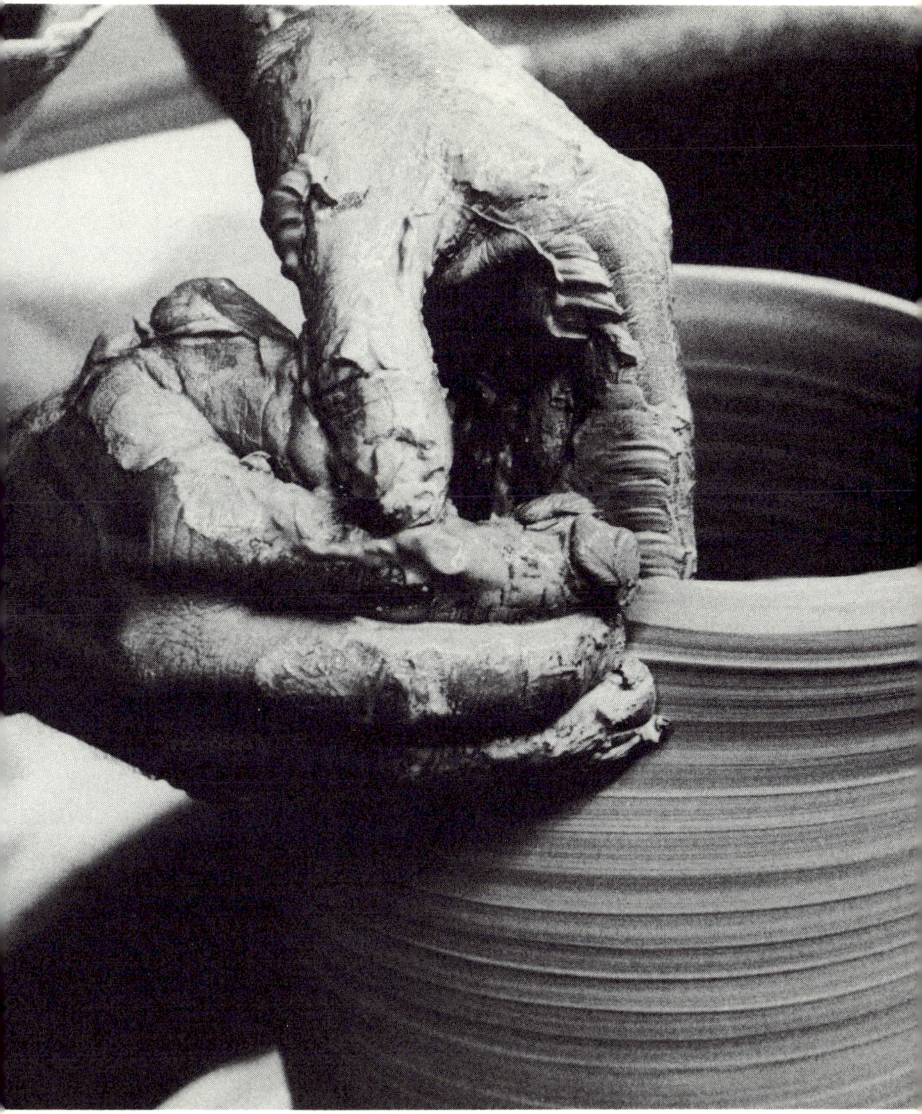

LIFE EXCERPT

Meeting Our Child's Serious Condition

"When the doctor told us our child's diagnosis, I began to feel sick to my stomach. I was really in shock. Me—a pastor who often was comforting somebody else." As Frank, a handsome man in his 30s, spoke, he glanced at his wife Marcia who sat nearby. Tears filled her eyes while he continued.

"After a few minutes with the doctor, I just had to excuse myself. I headed, shaking, for the men's room. I needed to be alone to get over the initial shock. When I got there, I stared into the mirror and saw a numb man. Then reality hit: This was happening to *me*, to my family. Then I told myself, 'With God's help you can make it through the consultation with the doctor.' And I did. I went back to be with my wife, to comfort her, and to go on from there."

These parents had been told that their six-year-old son had one of the forms of muscular dystrophy, and would probably not live to adulthood. They knew well what the condition could do. Marcia's brother had died fighting the clutches of that debilitating disease.

"After the first hours of learning of Robert's condition," Frank said, "we were a little more ourselves. Immediately both of us relied on our faith in the Lord. It was part of us. We talked a lot. We prayed together. And we talked about various scriptural promises that had been integrated into our lives."

They focused on God's larger perspective as recorded in Romans 8:28, "We know that in all things

God works for the good of those who love him, who are called according to his purpose."

"We reasoned that we'd keep our vision on eternity," Marcia explained. "And we want to set such a climate that we can be sure Robert will someday reach a point of 'being in Christ' as he lives on this earth." Both parents said they believed that if their children chose Jesus as Savior and Lord, they would experience the abundant life on both sides of eternity.

Marcia added, "We went through an initial grief period like so many other parents, I'm sure. Grief wasn't new, because before Robert, we lost a baby just a few hours after birth. At times we tend not to talk about our feelings, and things get worse. I get bottled up inside. There's tension in the family, and the special harmony in our marriage is hindered. So we've learned to keep talking things over."

Soon after Robert's diagnosis, Frank confided in the senior pastor with whom he works. "I wept as I told him the diagnosis," Frank recalled. "He was very compassionate, but he asked me some pointed questions to be sure I wasn't carrying unnecessary guilt."

One question was, "Do you believe Robert is this way because of punishment for your sins?" Frank could honestly say no, basing his thoughts on John 9:1-12, in which Jesus was asked, "Who sinned, this man or his parents, that he was born blind?" (verse 2). Jesus' answer was, "Neither this man nor his parents sinned, but this happened so that the work of God might be made displayed in his life." Frank and Marcia did not believe God caused their son's condition; rather, that it was part of living in a world in which evil plays a major role.

Frank explained that, as parents, they were constantly providing ways Robert could grow in intellectual skills and interests. "We want him to be useful and as independent as possible," he said. "I talk to him more and more about the weakness in his legs, letting him know there are many other avenues of endeavor. One of Marcia's and my main prayers is: Lord, what do you want us to do in raising our son that will glorify you in spite of his handicap?"

"We want Robert to live to the fullest," added Marcia, "but should he die before adulthood, we want him to have lived as an individual with a purpose on this earth—one that no one else can fulfill. We are also trying to build his self-esteem any way we can."

"I remember our first trips to the clinic with Robert," Frank reflected. "I felt such a comradeship—an unspoken fellowship—with the other parents in the waiting room. I knew they must hurt like I did." At times like that Frank's dependence on God deepened. "We speak of being in the fellowship of God," he continued. "Those are mystical words, but so many times I've really felt God's presence."

"Our local fellowship in the church has touched us so much too," added Marcia, citing the many times friends at church took them aside, clasped their hands, and assured them of their prayers.

"You can just sense their genuine love!" Frank said. "It's great to be with Christians like that."

A few of their church friends, on the other hand, had approached them with inappropriate advice or simplistic statements like, "Just ask God to heal him." Frank and Marcia were praying for Robert's healing, they emphasized, but working closely with the physicians, too.

"I can see how God uses people more and more," Frank concluded. "When we're with the doctor, he has such an air of confidence, it gives us courage."

The doctor gave them a key approach to living every day with their son: "Do everything possible to make it a meaningful day for him."

In that spirit, Frank and Marcia said they sought creative ways to feed Robert's mind and spirit. They played games as a family, sometimes rolling on the floor in gleeful wrestling. They went places together. And even though both parents worked, family time was a priority.

Frank had taken on some goals he didn't have before, including an extra job in general aviation. "I want to provide fully for Robert's needs that may be up the road," he explained. "His condition has taught me not to take any of our four kids for granted. So in the summer I often take a couple of the children along to my work—just to be together."

As these parents watched Robert play or carry out assigned jobs around the house, they saw a happy, outgoing boy. Although they knew more difficult times lay ahead, they chose to savor the good, meaningful days with hearts full of thanksgiving.

"In all these things we are more than conquerors through him who loved us" (Rom. 8:37).

PRAYERS

The Blow—It's Serious

Jesus, *please come*, whoever you are, wherever you are, *please come!* I don't know what else to pray. All I know is that a doctor has given us a big blow. We have a seriously ill child.

I'm not ready, Lord. "I'm still in shock. I can't believe this is happening to our family.

Just take me as I am, Lord, in all my confusion, in all my anger. Yes, *anger*. I'm angry at you for letting this happen to us. And I want to fight back at something; I want to fight for the well-being of our child! I feel I could do anything to win health for this precious one I love so much.

I stop in this moment of stillness, and I know deep inside that the battle is not mine to win. It's beyond me. It's very complicated. I realize most of all that you did not send this trouble. It is part of the evil in our imperfect world. O dear Lord, direct my energies as a parent, and don't let me crumble.

Please bless our child with your great love. Take us all into your everlasting arms right now, and uphold us in the days ahead.

"The Lord himself goes before you and will be with you; he will never leave you nor forsake you. Do not be afraid; do not be discouraged" (Deut. 31:8).

Facing a Child's Pain

Lord, the agony of seeing our child racked by pain is unbearable! I ran for a nurse, only to find out it was too soon for another pain shot. My own body aches in reaction. I can hold a small hand, but little more. Lord, please have mercy.

In this moment alone with you, I plead for your power! Do something, work through somebody, but touch this helpless one as only you can.

As I've learned more to listen to you, I turn my ears to you. What do you want to tell me?

O dear God, it kills me to see this suffering. Maybe that's it—*my* fighting for our child needs killing. I need to stop depending on my human strength, and admit my weakness before you. Then you can more fully live within me. Strengthen us all this very hour. I'm counting on it.

"But he said to me, 'My grace is sufficient for you, for my power is made perfect in weakness.' Therefore I will boast all the more gladly about my weaknesses, so that Christ's power may rest on me" (2 Cor. 12:9).

Unconditional Love

In choosing to belong to Christ
one becomes entwined
with the gentle cords
of God's endless love.
So bound, one becomes free
to give to the hurting,
to work with the needy
—with "no strings attached."

LIFE EXCERPT

Learnings from a Son's Permanent Condition

One of the faith-building parts of preparing this book was encountering parents with a story to tell when I least expected to. It was an answer to a frequent prayer: "Lord, show me the way to the people you want me to meet, those who have something special to share with other parents." He did.

On one occasion I was in a children's hospital to meet with the chaplain. I stopped in the snack shop. As I munched on a sandwich, I noticed a mother and father tenderly feeding their son in a wheelchair. A conversation began between us, and I knew that I was in the right place at the right time.

When I explained my writing project, they were very receptive. As they talked with me, I watched their handicapped son groan and pull on his mother's arms. Gordon was 15, mentally retarded to the extent that he could not talk, and plagued by physical disabilities, including cerebral palsy.

Mitch and Gladys spoke openly of their frustrating pilgrimage from doctor to doctor since Gordon was a baby. They had seen him through four major operations. Then his care became too much for them, and he now lived in a hospital many miles from home. His parents were torn between going to see him, and giving time to their other children.

"What keeps you going?" I asked. "Faith in each other and in God," Gladys replied without hesitation.

As she gently fed pieces of a Twinkie to her hungry boy, she told how one medical problem after another had appeared in Gordon's life.

"It was extremely difficult to find the right specialists," she said. "But I kept asking and going to get help! And Gordon's situation taught me patience that things aren't going to happen overnight. Seeing some doctors even turned out to be a dead end."

Mitch often accompanied Gladys and Gordon to see specialists. He explained the drain on the family, but then his face brightened. "One doctor told us he had never had a patient as loving as Gordon. He really gets his love across, even though he doesn't talk." The father's eyes turned misty as he added, "That's just about the greatest thing anyone can say about a person's kid."

Both parents radiated a tremendous affection for their son who is able to come home only on weekends. They believe that God allowed Gordon's afflictions for some reason—perhaps to teach people compassion.

Gladys cited the kind support of people in their church, especially a friend who also has a handicapped son. "We talk a lot. It really helps, because she understands."

"What would you encourage other parents of children with difficult medical problems to do?" I asked.

"I'd stand behind them, and support them," Gladys said. "Parents' groups are good. It's important to get into those. And I'd tell them, 'Don't let your spirit be emptied by doctors.' "

Both parents affirmed that God *will* be with those who are going through any trying situation.

When I spoke to Gordon and patted him on the shoulder, I sensed his warm spirit even though he could not respond verbally. As I clasped hands with his dedicated parents, and studied their kind faces, I admitted to myself that I had seen only a glimpse of their ongoing courage.

"The Lord's unfailing love surrounds the man who trusts in him" (Ps. 32:10).

PRAYERS

A Doctor's Perception

Lord, sometimes the hardest part is watching a doctor silently examine our child, searching the mysteries of his illness. A hush falls over the room, and I know you are right here with us. But, Lord, my inner ache rises to a throbbing pain to see our child suffering—and an effective treatment has not yet been found! I want to scream out, "When will all this be over for our family?"

Instead I fidget with my watch while he talks. He says he wants to "try something new" for treatment. It's a big risk. I tremble to think of it.

Dear God, I pray that you will grant your wisdom to the dedicated doctors who care for our child and many other young patients. Give them eyes to see what you want them to see and ears to hear what you want them to hear. Intervene in their perception—sometimes hazy—by the guidance of your Holy Spirit. Lead them in ways that will bring healing and protection to these hurting dear ones.

No more fidgeting for me, God. I'm going to stretch out my empty hands to you—in trust.

"Trust in the Lord with all your heart, and lean not on your own understanding; in all your ways acknowledge him, and he will make your paths straight" (Prov. 3:5-6).

The Great Physician

Creator of us all, I watch our child bravely resist this thing that threatens to overtake him. I'm not sure how to pray. This is all so new to me, but I trust you. I know that Jesus spent much of his ministry on this earth healing the sick, those with injury, and even those at death. In a sense, I shove through the crowd and bring *our child* to the Great Physician right now! In my own way and in the Spirit of Christ, I pray specifically. . . .

Lord, I believe you bring wholeness in many different ways. Perhaps you will begin with the inner being of this suffering one—a renewal of spirit, mind and emotions. Touch us all, Lord, and help us to set a good climate for healing, one of deep trust in what you can do. Help us to live in calmness and acceptance.

Thank you, O Lord, for all you are doing for our child this very hour. I praise your holy name!

"This is the assurance we have in approaching God: that if we ask anything according to his will, he hears us. And if we know that he hears us—whatever we ask—we know that we have what we asked of him" (1 John 5:14-15).

Part Two

Be Not Dismayed, for I Am Your God

Along Our Way

We struggle in confusion;
sometimes in dark unrest,
when solemn perplexities
stretch across our path.

But there is One who sees
beyond our painful steps,
and preserves our going out
and our coming in.

Abiding in him, we find
limitless power and
immeasurable love
truly coloring our trek.

The wonder of God's
closeness seeps into the depths
of our troubled beings
as we hear his words:
"Be not dismayed—
I am your God."

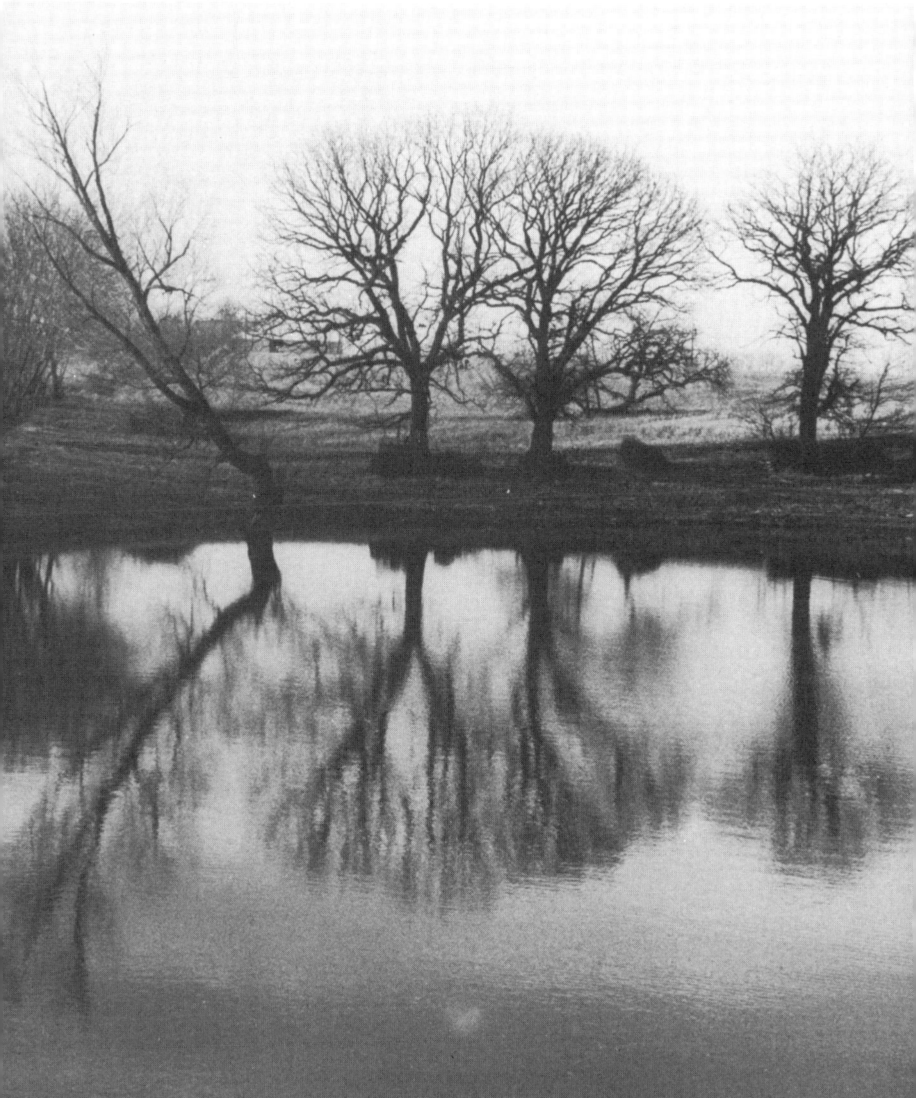

LIFE EXCERPT

A Daughter's Rehabilitation from an Accident

One phone call piercing a midnight in August changed everything in the lives of Marshall and Susan. They were told that their teen-aged daughter Lynn and some of her friends had been injured in a terrible car accident. Whirling in emotional terror and shock, these parents rushed to the hospital.

"I knew in my heart it was bad," Susan remembers. And indeed, Lynn was in critical condition, having suffered head injury and serious multiple injuries. She did not even know her parents; she was in a coma.

Susan remained at Lynn's side throughout the many weeks of crisis. Meanwhile, hundreds of people were praying.

"I felt if I left her," says Susan, "she wouldn't make it. A mother's instinct, I guess. At the same time, I quickly realized I couldn't operate in my own strength, so I grasped God's hand the best I knew how."

Lynn's progress was measured by the movement of a hand or a leg. Her family witnessed the power of prayer as she responded in delicate ways. After many weeks she regained consciousness. Yet Lynn was still in serious condition, and unable to talk.

Then, as though the gentle winds of God's Spirit had caught the sails of her threatened life, she began to move forward inch by inch in recovery. After two months in the hospital, she was transferred to a local rehabilitation center.

One of the hardest parts for Marshall and Susan was remembering how Lynn used to be—a bubbly teenager, a happy Christian girl, active in Young Life. Now doctors were telling them a grim prognosis: that they didn't expect her ever to recover enough to walk or talk, and that, very likely, she would have to be institutionalized the rest of her life. It was almost too much to bear.

Nevertheless, Susan recalls days at the rehabilitation center: "Everyone employed by that hospital became emotionally involved with Lynn and our family. It was like a day-by-day TV program, sending out reports to everyone. And anyone who didn't believe in miracles, anyone who worked around her, eventually changed his way of thinking. There was a love that emanated from Lynn to everyone who came into her room, whether they were nurses, physicians, or the cleaning women."

Progress continued. By December Lynn was flown to an excellent rehabilitation center in another state. Susan was allowed to stay at the center after she proved she wouldn't interfere with the therapy and coddle Lynn too much. During all of Lynn's hospitalizations, Susan was faced with many difficult decisions.

"You have to keep your wits about you," she says of that time. "You have to realize doctors are human; they make mistakes. I demanded to be told everything that would be done to our daughter. I had to meditate to ask God to guide me in all decisions.

"You also have to turn your complete will over to God," Susan adds thoughtfully. "There's nobody else who can help you in that life-or-death situation. Take just one day at a time. Sometimes you'll be able to handle just five minutes. But continue to believe that God is at work in each minute. If you don't believe, keep affirming in your own mind that God will do what is best."

By mid-February, some six months after her accident, Lynn was dismissed from the rehabilitation center. "On the day we left," Susan recalls, "the supervisory nurse surprised me with a beautiful orchid. It was very meaningful to me after all that had happened. It gave me more confidence in myself."

Lynn now lives at home, but she is quiet and struggling. Nurses and therapists assist her during periodic visits. She speaks slowly, in the monotone common to head-injured patients. Yet when she talked with me at the time of this interview, she spoke of her wonderful parents and of God's love. I, too, could feel love emanating from her. It showed me that the Christian spirit can triumph over injury, brain damage, or any physical disability.

Susan has no idea how much more her daughter will eventually recover, but she stresses, "We have years and years of rehabilitation ahead of us." Even so, at this point, Lynn is walking with aid. She can sit at a table and play an easy game.

"All these are miracles," Susan says, "because they are directly opposed to what I had been told all along the way. She can walk. She can talk. We are daily praising God!"

Susan is realistic about the future. "Even if Lynn has a hundred percent recovery, we'll never have our daughter back as she was prior to the accident. We'll have a daughter, but not the same personality. We had to teach her to smile. She doesn't laugh or cry, although she does show periods of anger. It is progress. She'll look at me and say, 'Can you tell I'm crying?' Well, that just breaks my heart."

Exhausted much of the time, Susan has experienced a drain on her health during constant care of Lynn. It has hardly been all victory. "Trouble comes when I try to get in the driver's seat and run things myself," she confides. "I actually forget God in those moments. It doesn't work."

Susan points to what sustains her most: worship with other Christians in church, her prayer life, her closeness to family and friends. She admits that she has not always been close to people. But many of those she came to know after Lynn's accident were so open toward her that she, in turn, took the risk to be open with them. These new friends and other parents helped her keep her perspective.

Marshall and Susan have often talked about their perspective since Lynn began to recover. "I never hesitate to say to anybody," declares Susan, "whether they're agnostic or Christian or whatever, that God has handled this. God has brought Lynn this far, and he won't drop her now."

Susan does not blame God for the accident, although she's not sure why it happened. "If it occurred for a reason," she reflects, "I feel it is the spreading of God's Word, because that's what has happened." Many people have witnessed God's reality and power through Lynn's situation.

The wonders of God's Word touched Susan's life several months after the accident. She began searching for a closer relationship with God. As part of that search, she attended a prayer group at her church. "I got to only one meeting," she says, "but what I felt there was a lot of love. I was touched spiritually like nothing I'd ever felt before. The presence of the Holy Spirit was very real, and verses from the Bible seemed meant just for me that day. I think the experience went a long way in helping me to trust God more fully. It didn't stop there, because members of that group came to the hospital and prayed and offered loving support."

Since that time, Susan can confidently say, "I have *really* sensed God's personal love for me. I believe I have come through all this because he carried me. And I know he carried Lynn and the rest of our family, too."

Lynn is now walking with the use of a cane, and has improved in overall coordination. She returned to public school, and took classes with other students who are disabled. Nearly four years after the accident, she has graduated from high school—an incredible feat.

At Lynn's commencement, she walked unaccompanied across the stage. She let go of her cane to shake hands with the school administrator, and to clasp the diploma. Immediately the crowd broke into a moving standing ovation. Her parents wept. For wonderful intense moments, a spirit of triumph hung over the stadium.

Since that time Lynn's mother has become active in the National Head Injury Foundation, and has helped to start chapters in two states.

PRAYERS

Where Is the Miracle?

Lord God, I'm hurt. I feel very let down. So many of our family and friends have joined me in praying for a miracle. We've met only your silence. My child's condition is hardly improved. Where is the miracle?

How can things be at such a standstill, Lord? I've stood on your scriptural promises, I've affirmed your power to heal, I've asked for thorough forgiveness, and I've even pleaded in prayer.

Silence.

Could it be that you are still entering into our situation, even though I see no supernatural acts? Yes, I believe you *are* working, because I know you as my heavenly Father. Surely you have larger, longer, and deeper purposes than I can see. I need to start looking for your little miracles, like more love and growth in each of us; like renewed strength when we thought we couldn't go on.

Teach me what to look for, O God, while I look for the big miracle. I know you love us with an everlasting love, and even in silence, you hold us in the palm of your hand. Deep, deep within I want *your will* for our child who thrives in your keeping.

"Call to me and I will answer you and tell you great and unsearchable things you do not know" (Jer. 33:3).

"Now faith is being sure of what we hope for and certain of what we do not see" (Heb. 11:1).

When Needing More Faith

I am often reminded of other people's wonderful faith in you, the living God. Secretly I wish I could be more like them. They show radiance, confidence, trust. Sometimes I even pretend to be a strong believer, but I'm not fooling anyone, especially you. I'm seized with fear when I think of what could happen to our child as he fights a terrible illness. And fear is the opposite of faith! O dear God, guide my thoughts toward you, toward your love and power. Cast out my fear. We desperately need you!

I'm trying to turn to the Scriptures more often. One day I read that you give each believer a measure of faith. That spoke to me. Perhaps you just want me to be myself, and to draw on insights from your Word. As I step out on your gift of faith, will you supply more? I'm beginning to realize you will.

Lord, I recall a conversation with our dedicated pastor. He spoke of his focus through a favorite verse: "Let us fix our eyes on Jesus, the author and perfecter of our faith" (Heb. 12:2). I have been looking too much to people. More looking to Jesus!

"Faith comes from hearing the message, and the message is heard through the word of Christ" (Rom 10:17).

"I tell to you the truth, if you have faith as small as a mustard seed . . . nothing will be impossible for you" (Matt. 17:20).

Praise for Progress

Lord, you amaze me
in the surprise way
you answer prayer.

Your wisdom is beyond
my tiny understanding.

I hoped you would heal
our hurting child
with a swoop of your hand.

Instead you shed
sweet new light
upon our daily living.

You taught us to pour
love into one another;
to listen in tenderness.

Lord, I praise you
for the steady progress
in the one for whom
we prayed—
one who dwells in
a love-filled home.

LIFE EXCERPT

A Mother's Flashback

by Esther L. Vogt

It was Saturday, December 10, 1949. Long hours of pain finally climaxed when the miracle of birth was over. My heart sang, for we had a son and Shirley had her baby brother. But our joy was short-lived as Dr. Janzen faced us solemnly.

"Your baby is very ill," he said. "Due to the difficult delivery he suffered brain damage. It's just a matter of time. . . . "

I stared dismally at the brightly lit Christmas tree that stood at the south end of the corridor on the first floor of the old hospital building, its lights blinking off and on. I felt like stopping my ears as the sound of carols drifted up and down those red-bricked walls: "Joy to the world. . . . " How dared they sing of joy when, for us, all joy had drained away?

Shirley told her Sunday school teacher that Sunday morning, "I have a new baby brother, but I think he's going to be with Jesus for Christmas."

On Monday the nurse rustled into my room. She laid the blanketed bundle into my arms without a word. I suppose they thought he would soon be gone, so I might as well hold him while I had the chance.

As the baby whimpered and moaned, my tears dripped down the wizened, pain-wracked face. I couldn't bear my own helplessness to help him, and I cried: "Dear God, take him!"

Half an hour later I rang for the nurse. "I can't bear it," I told her. "Please take him away." I prayed only that it might be over soon. Each time the nurse came into my room I wanted to shake her for news of Ranney, but she didn't volunteer any information, and I couldn't bring myself to ask.

On Tuesday morning Dr. Janzen stepped into my room and seated himself on the edge of my bed. He seemed excited.

"I don't know what's happened, Esther," he said, "but your baby is very much better today. We're feeding him with a medicine dropper. He's still very weak, but the fever is down. I think he'll make it."

I went home several days before Christmas, although Ranney had to remain in the hospital nursery. We visited him every day. At first we were allowed to watch him only through the nursery window. Then one day the nurse wheeled him into an empty room. I noticed the splints on both arms. We learned that although he would be physically handicapped, his mind was sharp and keen. (Today he's a college honor graduate, who in spite of cerebral palsy, holds down a good job in Emporia, Kansas.)

On Christmas Day Curt and I took Shirley along on our daily visit to the hospital. The nurse picked up Ranney from the crib and laid him in my arms.

"Here," she said, handing the bottle to me. "Feed him. He's graduated from the medicine dropper to the bottle."

I noticed the bandage was already off one arm. All trace of pain was gone from the round little face, which was now colored a delicate normal pink.

Shirley brushed the tiny cheeks with her fingers. "Merry Christmas, baby brother," she said softly.

And this time, as the carols floated down the hall, I hummed along.

Esther Vogt, now an author of a number of books, stories and articles, adds a few comments about raising a child with cerebral palsy.

Ranney was always cheerful and optimistic, making it easy to run through the routine of tedious exercising. There were times when my own patience almost failed and I thought he'd never learn. But I knew that he had to persist if he were to learn any degree of independence when he grew up.

Not everyone understood our insistence that he do things for himself. After many trials and errors, he finally learned to get up by himself after his frequent falls. It wasn't easy to watch him struggle to his feet alone, and I often ached to rush to his aid. One day after he had fallen at the post office, I stood by patiently as he pulled himself to his feet. Later, someone told one of my friends that I was a "cruel" mother. Poor Ranney had fallen down and I had refused to help him up!

Most of all, raising Ranney took daily prayers and dedication. I was continually asking for the Lord's wisdom and direction and especially patience when Ranney became frustrated. Yet the Lord never let us down. His grace was always sufficient, just as he has promised.

"I will extol the Lord at all times; his praise will always be on my lips. My soul will boast in the Lord; let the afflicted hear and rejoice. Glorify the Lord with me; let us exalt his name together" (Ps. 34:1-3).

PRAYERS

Another Parent

Thank you, Lord, for allowing me to meet another parent who shares a parallel pilgrimage. We were drawn together in sincere caring for one another's situation. How marvelous to be able to share freely with another—one who really understands, one whose eyes say, "I've been there, too."

Surely you will bless this new relationship, Lord. Help me to do my part to listen intently and be a timely friend. I pray now for this parent and the child who needs your healing and sustaining touch. May your love be very real to each member of that family. Show me ways in which I can reach out to my new friend.

Again I praise you for your wonderful ways in my life. You must have a beautiful plan to have brought us parents together at this point in our trying journey. Our sense of kinship and mutual support will surely be a lift to us in the days ahead.

"Encourage one another and build each other up, just as in fact you are doing" (1 Thess. 5:11).

Home from the Hospital

It is so good, God, to have our child home from the hospital! We thank you for the steady improvement.

Excitement and joy rippled through me to see our child's face beam as we entered our house. The aroma of homemade soup, the melody of a favorite record playing, and most of all being together, have contributed to fresh color in our child's cheeks.

Now that we are settled into familiar surroundings, I actually feel a little let down—an indescribable void. I realize I'm missing the hospital staff we came to know so well. They pulled together in a mighty tug-of-war against that which is hurting our child. They seemed like family. They were tuned into what concerned us most—every symptom, every change. They showed they cared. I miss their timely words and ready smiles. Bless those doctors, nurses, and aides—bless them all.

Thank you for their team effort so close behind us. Now help me, God, to count on you as my close companion as I care for our child in the days ahead.

"And surely I will be with you always, to the very end of the age" (Matt. 28:20).

Part Three

Times of Prayer

Comfort

O Lord, my soul is heavy,
my heart bowed down.
I seek the gentle Comforter
to touch my hidden hurts.
Being uplifted again by your mercy,
I become a channel of love
to those who hurt
even more.

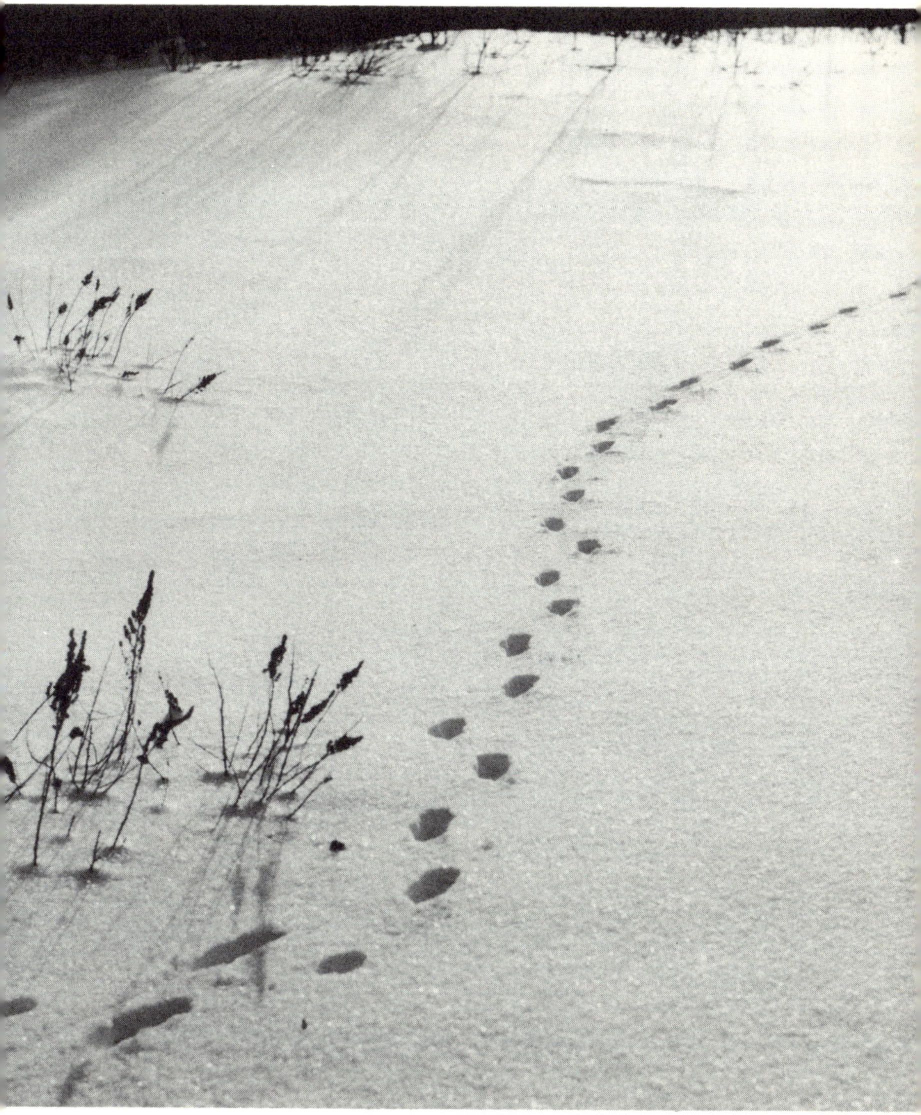

PRAYERS

I'm Not Religious

I have just enough faith to call you God. You know I'm not religious, never having talked to you much. If you are the living God people preach about, can you hear me now? *Someone* has to hear me!

We have a very sick child who may not live more than two years. I've been numb; now I grieve. I feel lost in a wilderness of medical battle for that life!

I see other parents at the hospital, bowing their heads in prayer when their pastor comes. Sometimes they appear to have all the answers. They believe you will act in some marvelous way, because the Bible says so. Will you?

A friend told me, "I really believe God meets us where we are in our need." Here's *our* need, God! Look it over. It's too much for us. I want to think you will meet us some way.

I don't even know any Bible verses—just "The Lord is my shepherd. . . . " I whisper to you now. Will you be my Shepherd in this wilderness? I'm taking steps toward you. Please lead me to those still waters. Restore my hurting soul. Most of all, if possible, restore our child.

"He who comes to me will never go hungry, and he who believes in me will never be thirsty. But as I told you, you have seen me and still you do not believe. All that the Father gives me will come to me, and whoever comes to me I will never drive away" (John 6:35-37).

More than "the Blues"

Heavenly Father, I really need you. I fear I'm falling apart, right when my husband and children need me most. I'm exhausted from not sleeping. Food seems to stick in my throat, and I'm avoiding people.

When I talked with our pastor, his eyes met mine with compassion, but his words penetrated me: "You are in a heavy depression." He helped me to see that too much anger and fear and self-pity are stored inside me. O dear God, can *that* happen to a Christian? It has. Please have mercy!

Wash out my crippling anxiety, my self-pity, all through the power of Christ. Forgive me for absorbing negative, fearful thoughts instead of relying on your Holy Spirit, my closest Counselor. I want to center on you as I face *all* of the daily distresses of having a sick child.

And dear God, I know your spirit is ever-present. If need be, give me the humility to talk out my anguish with a trained human counselor. Lead me to someone who seeks your guidance, too.

"Heal me, O Lord, and I will be healed; save me, and I will be saved, for you are the one I praise" (Jer. 17:4).

When the Burden Is Heavy

Lord, I come in utter stillness to this lovely park to be alone with you. I'm drained. I want to absorb the beauty and strength of your creation all about me. It's a relief to leave behind my rushing, the smell of a hospital, the ringing phone. In silence I sense your presence. You understand. You know I'm all knotted up inside, trying not to cry. Thank you for your constant compassion that seems to wrap itself around my suffering child and around me.

O dear God, I can't hold back any longer! I'm tired of "being strong" in front of everyone. Tears burn my eyes and, with all my heart, I *give you this burden* of a sick child. And I pause in silent trust to listen to you. . . .

Thank you, God. It all feels lighter now. You carry the load.

"In quietness and trust is your strength" (Isa. 30:15).

Cast your cares on the Lord and he will sustain you" (Ps. 55:22).

My Irritability

A gray sadness hangs over me, heavenly Father, when I think of how irritable I've been today. I even sent one of our children crying to her room, because I yelled at her for no good reason. Little things are getting to me. I'm ashamed of the way I've acted. O dear God, please forgive me.

Lord, give me the grace to be in control of my actions and emotions, especially during this time of stress with a sick child. My family needs me at my best. I don't want to hurt sensitive lives anymore. Fill me, Lord, with what it takes.

As I ponder all that is going on in our household, I think of what a dear friend said: "You have a tough situation. It's OK to blow off steam once in a while. Your family can take it." May our love be big enough to accept one another as we are, just as you accept us through Christ. I'm learning, Lord, I'm learning.

"Love bears all things, believes all things, hopes all things, endures all things" (1 Cor. 13:7 RSV).

Telephone Temptation

Dear God, our child recently set me straight with, "Mom, you're *always* on the phone." It's true.

Too often I've attached myself to a telephone cord and left my husband and children to dangle in their needs. I've even neglected our ill child at times to talk on the phone. Please forgive me, God.

And please forgive me for praying to you expectantly one minute, and then telling a friend who calls how bad things are the next. I confess I'm wanting sympathy. Worst of all, the whole family has overheard my negative talk!

It's time for me to take some giant steps in growing up, just as our child has done. He doesn't talk about the hurting; he lives resiliently for the moment. In childlike faith, he trusts you.

I thank you, Lord, for kind support from friends. It has its place. Surely you don't want me to thrive on people's sympathy, but on your love and care. Help me in these daily choices.

"May the words of my mouth and the meditation of my heart be pleasing in your sight, O Lord, my Rock and my Redeemer" (Ps. 19:14).

What Shall I Read?

Lord, while our child grows weaker in a hospital room, I'm groping for hope, for answers.

When the doctor saw me in the hall, he spotted the books I held, one in each hand. One focused on miracles; the other was *On Death and Dying.*

"You'd better read *that* one," he said firmly, pointing to the word dying. His comment stabbed me!

Dear God, I'm all confused. Is the doctor being cruel or wise? Perhaps I *do* need to understand the stages of coping that our child is moving through. I want to be close to him in this crisis, heart to heart. It would tear me up to find out that he unburdened his feelings to a nurse because we, his parents, fled from his life-threatened world.

Guide me in what to read during the long hours while our child sleeps. Most of all, help me to absorb the wisdom and power and hope in your Word. I want to read other material in the context of your Spirit—and discover my needed tools. And Lord, I'm going to keep focusing on you in the muddle of advice beckoning from all sides. I want to grope less and grasp more to your mighty hand. Help me.

"I will instruct you and teach you in the way you should go; I will counsel you and watch over you" (Ps. 32:8).

As a Single Parent

I'm a "survivor," God, of an ended marriage, and the continuous challenge of raising children. Some days I feel absolutely trapped in the round-the-clock demands of my handicapped child. I confess I resent doing things for someone—all of the time.

I don't like being single. It's an aching strain. Dear God, I fear facing the deterioration of my child's condition alone. We *all* need you as Helper in our household.

My children mean more to me than ever. I want to fulfill my role as parent in a beautiful way. But I don't feel beautiful. I want to take in your Spirit more deeply to fill the crevices of my hollow self. How else can I really meet the love commitment to these children?

Lord, my situation could have been devastating, but you blessed my efforts. I'm grateful. And I never would have made it without my friends! Thank you for using them to help me feel better about myself. Bless them richly.

"Consider it pure joy, my brothers, whenever you face trials of many kinds, because you know that the testing of your faith develops perseverance. Perseverance must finish its work so that you may be mature and complete, not lacking anything" (James 1:2-4).

To Forgive Others

People seem to let me down, Lord, just when I need them most. Friends I thought I could count on don't even bother to call. Our doctor makes a careless mistake in a prescription causing an upset in our child's already sick body. A relative criticizes the way we are "spoiling" our child. Even our sick child makes great demands on my time, sometimes with whims. They all make me angry, and anger tends to harden into resentment. I'm ashamed.

Please help me, Lord, to fully forgive each of those who snag the smoothness and satisfactions I want in raising our child, one with unusual needs. Especially help me to understand that most people have about all they can carry, and they don't mean to let me down.

I recognize the impurities settling in my life. I need cleansing. I need *you*, God. Restore in me a forgiving heart, and a controlled tongue. May I never again speak cruelly of those whom I'm seeking to forgive. I draw on your loving grace in all my relationships.

"Therefore, as God's chosen people, holy and dearly loved, clothe yourselves with compassion, kindness, humility, gentleness and patience. Bear with each other and forgive whatever grievances you may have against one another. Forgive as the Lord forgave you. And over all these virtues put on love, which binds them all together in perfect unity" (Col. 3:12-14).

When a Child Suffers from Mental Illness

An overwhelming feeling of helplessness has fallen upon us, dear God. Our child's strange symptoms and behavior are now labeled a form of mental illness. Where can I go to scream?

I choose to get alone with you, God, and let out all that is bottled up. This is the worst agony I've ever suffered—to deal with a child who is losing contact with reality. Why didn't we see it sooner?

One minute we ache for him; the next we almost hate him! What messed-up parents we are. Oh, God, help us! Wash away any resentment and anger toward our child, and guide us into effective parenting. We need a daily dose of compassion. Forgive our heavy guilt, and touch us with your peace and hope. And, Lord, please help us not to blame each other.

I see I can't handle this situation. For the first time, I'm beginning to really depend on you. Lead us to the right specialists who will help us as a family to work through our many problems. We know *you* have the power to unlock our child's being, so that he can function as a whole person. We want to set a climate of positive living that will help his personality to blossom.

In faith I see our child's life being built on a rock that will crush the ugly vines of evil, threatening to entangle him. You are that rock!

"The Lord is my strength and my shield; my heart trusts in him and I am helped" (Ps. 28:7).

Before a Child's Surgery

It's very difficult for me, heavenly Father, to kiss our child, squeeze his little hand, and then to see him wheeled into an operating room. It is hard to let go. But I must.

In simple trust, I commit this one I love very much into your keeping. Please guide the minds and hands of skilled surgeons. Give alertness to persons administering anesthetics or giving aid in any way. I pray for *the best* for our child!

And, O Father, I cringe to think of the pain that could come after surgery. I pray for relief from such suffering. Please have mercy.

I see my child now, slipping into deep sleep for the operation, under the shadow of the Almighty! Thank you, Father, for hearing this prayer—a prayer for full victory and healing!

"He who dwells in the shelter of the Most High will rest in the shadow of the Almighty" (Ps. 91:1).

"Peace I leave with you; my peace I give you. I do not give to you as the world gives. Do not let your hearts be troubled, and do not be afraid" (John 14:27).

Finances to Figure

O Lord, our minds whirl as we examine the enormous unbelievable expenses for our child's medical care! We are thankful for insurance and help from caring agencies, yet our funds are being consumed by scores of other costs, too. It hurts. Each month it is a miracle how you provide financially. We truly thank you, and we trust you for the future.

Not every family is as blessed as we are, Father. I think of many others who have been shattered by gigantic medical costs.

I pray for a young couple I met at the hospital. Medical insurance hardly touches their bills. Their baby's condition doesn't qualify them for funds from any given group. And the tangle of our laws leaves them without aid. When I asked these parents if perhaps their church could hold a benefit, the mother just stared at me. "We've been unable to go to our new church," she said. "Then the pastor stopped coming to see us. We couldn't ask the church."

Where *are* Christians at a time like theirs? I pray someone will hear their cry. Show us all ways to help one another.

"Do not be anxious about anything, but in everything, by prayer and petition, with thanksgiving, present your requests to God. And the peace of God, which transcends all understanding, will guard your hearts and your minds in Christ Jesus" (Phil 4:6-7).

Help for a Sleepless Night

It's miserable, it's terrifying, Lord, not to be able to sleep. I finally climb out of bed to ease my tense muscles. I try exercises. I try to center on pleasant thoughts. Nothing works.

I can't understand this restlessness. I thought I had surrendered all my problems to you, but as I try to sleep, a nebulous anxiety grips me. I'm carrying the burdens of yesterday and the fears of tomorrow—our seriously ill child's tomorrow! Please show me the way to peace and rest.

Lord, I know you are nearer than hands and feet. Your love is very real. I'm going to write or whisper out loud to you my specific anxicties about our child. And here, Lord, are other heavy concerns. . . . Now I place *all* of my conscious and subconscious worries into your hands, trusting you will work on them even during the night.

Some people turn to the Scriptures when they can't sleep. I'll try that, too. I open to the Psalms, and uncover the heart cries of David—much like my own. And then I see his abounding praise to you. In my own patterns of silent praise and release, I slip back into bed.

"The eternal God is your refuge, and underneath are the everlasting arms" (Deut. 33:27).

"Cast all your anxiety on him because he cares for you" (1 Peter 5:7).

It's a New Day

A new day breaks upon us, Father. Before I slip out of bed, I whisper praise to you, our Creator. I offer myself anew in your service. Recreate me more and more in your image throughout the hours ahead.

Instead of the pain in my heart, I focus on your faithfulness as I hear birds singing outside, and my family stirring in another room. I sense the beckoning of your love as I make a fresh start.

I thank you for your enduring companionship, your grace, and your steadfast love—through *everything*.

Open my eyes to your wonders and your workings in the promise of this bright new day. Help me to shed negative thoughts, and to be filled with your Holy Spirit. I thank you for nurturing my growth over past months, to become more than just curious about you, but consecrated in your service as a parent. Keep working on me!

I recall the happy as well as the hurting days behind us. At times I thought I would collapse inside, but I hung on, discovering your promise: "Fear not, for I am with you." I see how your presence has enfolded us, your guidance has helped us, your power has strengthened us, and your mighty love through Christ has upheld us.

I adore you in glad song as I step out to savor with my family this new day, even with its troubles. You are at our side.

"It is good to praise the Lord and make music to your name, O Most High, to proclaim your love in the morning and your faithfulness at night" (Ps. 92:1-2).

In Search of a Rainbow

Reaching for magnificent roses,
we are scratched by thorns.
Searching for brilliant rainbows,
we are drenched by downpours.
Dreaming of vibrant health,
we are brought down by sickness.

May we journey with Christ Jesus
Who suffered Calvary's thorns,
Who walked on water,
Who healed the sick.
He is more than a rainbow—the One
Who transforms us in it all.

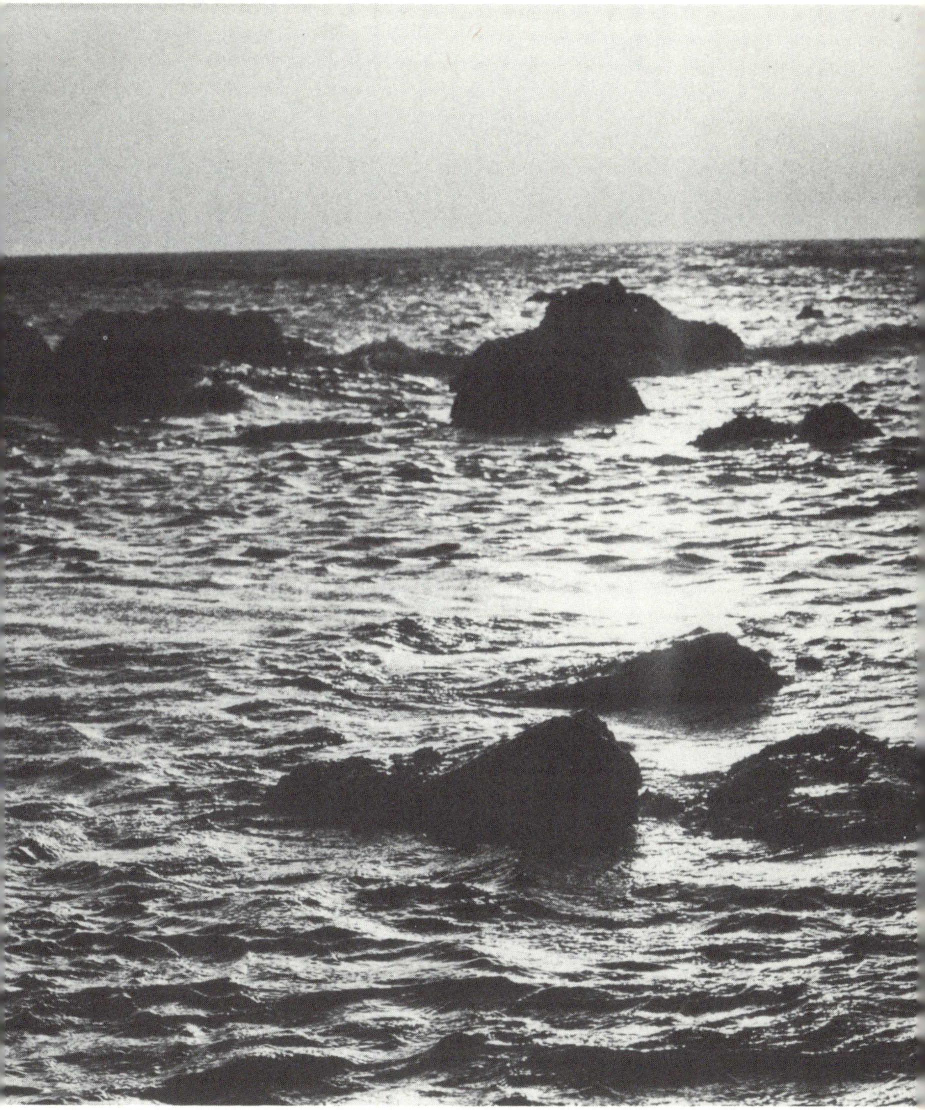

Part Four

I Will Strengthen You

A Secret of Strength

In prayerful moments
subtle peace comes
when I choose to drop
my fearful baggage
into Greater Arms.
Traveling lighter
I can move swiftly
with resilient response
to whatever happens.
As in a mystery—
I am filled with
new strength.

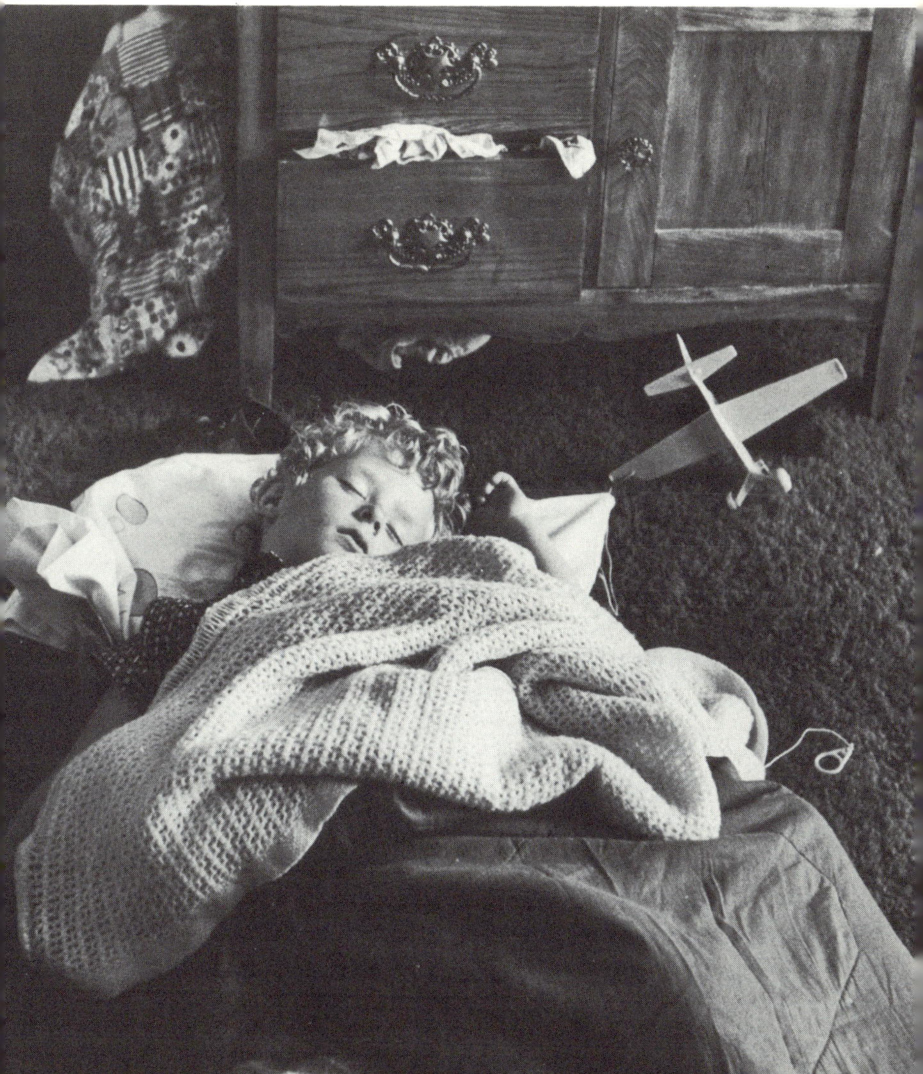

LIFE EXCERPT

A Sixth-Grader Copes from a Wheelchair

One of my privileges was coming to know 14-year-old Edward, a good student in a suburban elementary school. Daily he rolls his motorized wheelchair into his sixth-grade classroom, and meets the routine. He is a handicapped student who has been mainstreamed into the everyday world of public school.

As I observed Edward in the classroom, I concluded that he is hardly an "everyday" boy. Muscular weakness controls his life to the extent that he must be dressed by someone, assisted in a restroom, and lifted into bed. This type of muscular dystrophy, which he has had since age three, is progressive, so that Edward might not live through his teens.

Edward is held together by more than a back brace; he is motivated by an inner drive that grabs at the opportunities of each day. With determination he finishes each assignment, working at his slower rate at a special desk, constructed to fit his wheelchair.

Teachers speak of their fondness for him, and express their continuous admiration. Unfortunately, many classmates leave him in an isolated world. Some react by pretending he's not there.

"I don't like it when kids stare at me or make faces," Edward confides. "But God doesn't care what we look like or what mistakes we make. He loves us just the same. And he pays attention to us." Edward watches his squirming classmates while they work on a class project. "They just don't know how lucky they are to be healthy," he adds, his arms resting limply on his lap.

A highlight for Edward each week is attending a fellowship group for handicapped youth held at a local church, where he delights in camp-type songs and games. "I wouldn't miss it!" he says with a wide smile. He belongs.

Edward also feels a kinship with young people at the medical center. Many have similar conditions. "We all keep trying," he says. When asked about the good he sees in his situation and that of others at the center, he pauses. "The best thing I can say is, well, we're still alive, aren't we? What I mean is, I feel like I am part of a team with the other kids at the clinic. We're a fighting team. We're fighting to do our best with what we have."

Edward's mother adds her thoughts to Edward's. "It *is* an accomplishment for him to be alive," she affirms. "He doesn't really know the grim prognosis of muscular dystrophy, but he is aware he's going downhill. He's weaker. He's more melancholy. The sad thing is his emptiness. His loneliness. Edward is isolated from what a 14-year-old would be doing with other kids. Few kids know how to enter into a handicapped person's life. So we're giving Edward all the good experiences we can, even if it's just going to the library. And we do have fun! Life just isn't any good if you don't *live* it."

Richness of living is the accent of Edward's family life. His younger sister has been taught to help a lot so that they can do enjoyable things together. The family has adopted a motto to draw on in all frustrating situations: "Love is the important thing."

"At times, though," confides his mother, "I sit down and cry. I know the day will come when Edward will be confined to bed. And I must be prepared to . . . someday lose him. It's hard. Very hard. But on the practical side, I'm handling it only a few minutes at a time. And there is *always* hope that medical science will come through in time to help Edward."

When asked where she feels God is in their situation, she breaks into a smile. "God is very strong. He's *right here*."

"For you have been my hope, O Sovereign Lord, my confidence since my youth" (Ps. 71:5).

PRAYERS

Special Moments with Our Child

Heavenly Father, I think of so many happy moments with each member of our family. You have blessed us with an abundance of joys and satisfactions. Thank you!

I think especially of our child who continues to fight a life-threatening disease. I cherish those times when he took a walk with me or chatted as we rode in the car. I recall the silly moments when he teased me into being a child again, and we rolled on the floor with laughter.

Most special, Father, are those evenings when we share heart-to-heart talks. Once he asked, "What is God like?" and I told him something of your wondrous love. "Jesus showed us what God is like," I said.

Months later he shared that he had a new friend. "Who is your friend?" I asked. "Jesus," he answered with a broad, confident smile. O dear God, that smile must have reached your heart, too!

Every day this lovable, wonderful child is going to need more and more of your love and strength and closeness. When some dying children gaze at the TV for their only "outside" contact, I want our child to be offered more. I want to offer him myself, and I want him to have you. You are the One who will see him through everything—even through eternity.

"Teach them to your children, talking about them when you sit at home and when you walk along the road" (Deut. 11:19).

Our Other Children

Heavenly Father, I see it now. We've been so preoccupied with our hurting child that we've spun past our other children. I ache as I see increased misbehavior, frequent ailments and empty looks on their faces. They seem to be calling out, "Look at me, really look at me!" I realize now that our indifference to them can cause the deepest hurt of all.

Please forgive us, Father. We don't mean to slight any of our family. Help us to find time for each of our children, even though our days are so full of extra demands. We want to be good listeners and to be consistent in our love.

I pray specifically for our healthy children. Wash out any jealousy or resentment that may be taking root in them. May they know by the way we treat them that they are truly special. I go in your love now, O God, to look fully into the eyes of our children.

"A new command I give you: Love one another. As I have loved you, so you must love one another. All men will know that you are my disciples if you love one another" (John 13:34-35).

My Search

How long I sought a great cathedral
abounding with God's love
to enfold me!

I desired a mighty message
of his unique plan
to lift my aching heart.

Then a sacred place I found
where no anthems rang;
no brilliant light.

I felt a tiny hand in mine
in the hush of earnest prayer
around our family's table:

"Thank you, Lord, that
we all are gathered
here together."

A tender voice
filled a great cathedral.

LIFE EXCERPT

A Baby's Intensive Care

Every daytime hour, and sometimes at night, Carol donned a sterile gown and mask, and entered an isolated hospital room to cuddle her firstborn baby Matt. He broke into a smile each time he heard his mother's voice, even though he was attached to irritating tubes and medical equipment. All but three weeks of Matt's four months of life had been spent in the ICU—the Intensive Care Unit at a children's hospital where he had undergone numerous lifesaving surgeries.

Immediately after birth, Matt turned blue, gasping for air and choking when he exhaled. The doctors discovered that Matt's esophagus connected to his trachea—or windpipe—rather than to his stomach. Thus food and saliva pass abnormally from the esophagus to the trachea and into the lungs. This defect is one of the forms of T-E fistula, a continuous life-threatening condition. It often causes pneumonia. Matt was being treated nonstop with sophisticated medical equipment, emergency surgeries and his parents' fervent prayers.

Carol, an attractive 25-year-old brunette, took time to talk with me in the parents' lounge of the hospital, only minutes from her son's isolated chamber. She readily shared that she was emotionally drained and constantly anxious. "I swing from optimism to pessimism," she confessed. "Matt will seem better; then a new complication pops up, and it looks like we'll lose him."

When Carol and her husband, Howard, learned of their baby's critical problems, they were crushed. As Christians they began to ask God why. Carol had taken excellent care of herself during pregnancy. She had never smoked or used alcohol or drugs. It didn't seem fair. Nevertheless, "fair" or not, newborn Matt silently struggled for life. "I was so happy when I first heard him cry," she told me, "because for so long he never made a sound."

Many dark days fell on Carol and Howard. For several weeks it seemed Matt would not live, as he was rushed in and out of operating rooms and back into ICU. During that time Carol had the urge to phone her grandfather, a minister, and ask him, Is there *really* a God? But she never made the call. "I was really depressed," she explained. "Crises don't necessarily bring you closer to God at the time. Sometimes I was too upset to think of God."

The most significant helps for Carol were her husband, her pastor, several nurses who let themselves get involved, and other parents at the hospital. When one mother was ready to leave the hospital with her improved child, she looked into Carol's strained face and pleaded, "No matter what happens, don't let yourself withdraw. And don't ever give up hope."

Carol has tried to follow that mother's advice. She reaches out to others, and she has not given up hope. She does all she can to help answer her own prayers for Matt by giving him generous doses of love and body contact.

"It's most important that a child in ICU never go a day without mommy and daddy," she stressed. "He or she must have someone to live for. I've seen children die in the hospital— children who should have lived—because no parent showed up."

It strengthened Carol recently to find a new friend, another young mother who is often in the parents' lounge. "We cry with each other," Carol told me. "We sit up together at night when neither of us can sleep." Carol noticed that this mother quietly read her Bible every night. "That really impressed me," Carol commented. "She lives her faith in such a sweet, meaningful way. We both find it faith-building to remember times when we've seen God at work, and then think about those when times are dark."

Seven months after my visit with Carol, I talked with her again. Matt, now 11 months old, had lived most of his life in ICU. He had struggled through 13 surgeries—some successful, some not. His tissues had become chronically weak from all of the operations. Doctors had discovered another problem, too. The cartilage ring was missing from his trachea. Matt hit one crisis after another. When he was 10 months, a tracheotomy was performed, leaving an opening at his throat so he could vent better.

"Last month was really bad," Carol began. She caught her breath, and sobs broke her words. "Matt's heart stopped. That's when it really hit me—it could all be over. Fortunately, the doctor was right there, and gave him manual heart resuscitation. While they gave Matt oxygen, shivers went over me, and I realized God's power at work. I knew it wasn't only the doctor keeping him alive."

For several months the doctors had been telling Carol and Howard that they couldn't let Matt off oxygen; that he wouldn't live without it. But in time Matt rallied and was able to leave the oxygen tent.

"It was a big prayer answered," Carol said. "And when that happened, one of the doctors took us aside and said, 'The only reason your son is alive is that God wants him to live.' " Carol and Howard were moved by those words, and they gave God the glory.

Carol recognized she has gone through a sequence of stages in coping with life-and-death situations. Like other parents at the hospital, she tended to move back and forth into various stages. Never having heard lectures or read books about such stages, she openly described her spiritual journey in this way:

- You are shocked. You are crushed.
- You become "super-religious." You might pray all the time—sometimes frantically.
- Then you realize, hey, this isn't working out, and you get angry. One time I wanted to pound at God and yell, "I'm so *mad* at you!"
- Then you grieve. You might grieve off and on in any stage.
- Then you move into the apathy phase. You think God's not going to help. "What did I do to cause this?" jumps into your mind. When I thought this, I felt terribly alone.
- You move into the final stage. I'm there now. You come to the place where you face the reality that your child has serious problems. I guess you'd call it acceptance. You let God move back into the picture (even though he was there all along). For me,

> he's my companion. He's powerful, but he doesn't always work miracles. Many times I've sensed God's love. It's unconditional love; it comes no matter what I'm like at the time.

"When you just *have* to have relief from all the pain," Carol added, "God gives it. In our case, God sent us very special friends whom we met at the hospital. I see him working through these friends, and I hope he'll work through me as I try to support other parents.

"We became unusually close to Darrell and Ruby when their baby was also in ICU. We could sense their natural, built-in Christian faith. A beautiful bond grew between us, because we were going through our babies' touch-and-go situations together."

Darrell's and Ruby's 11-month-old baby died, but only three days after the funeral, they called Carol and Howard to see how Matt was. They came often to visit, and continued to give support.

"When Matt became extremely critical," related Carol, "Darrell came to see us at ICU, his first time back at the hospital. He stayed with us through an evening of anxiety, ache and exhaustion. His presence was very comforting. He sat in the very spot he'd been when his son died six months earlier. I don't know how he did it, except by the power of God in his life."

Matt is 20 months old now, and lives at home. Carol reports that he looks good, weighs 21 pounds, and is crawling. She says it's like running a hospital at home, charting, counting calories, using sophisticated machines and reporting to the doctor. Matt has to be connected to a machine to be fed a special formula that enters his intestines through intravenous tubes.

"Matt's situation is still extremely life-threatening," says Carol, "and it doesn't let up. One of us has to be with him at all times. Many times he stops breathing, and we administer resuscitation and oxygen. It's a terrible strain, but I can cite so many instances when God seemed to take over. Because of that my faith has deepened, and I keep remembering our doctor's words: God wants him to live."

Carol is planning for the future. Because Matt has no voice, he's learning some sign language. She is taking a course to learn sign language herself in order to teach him. She will do anything to help her lovable, fine looking boy. She admits, however, that at times she moved out of the acceptance stage when Matt got worse. She is honest and transparent; she still hurts deeply. During my last visit with her, we talked about Job of the Old Testament who progressed through unique spiritual stages as he dealt with agony, and ended up proclaiming, "I *know* that my Redeemer lives!" Carol can proclaim it, too.

Postscript: By age four Matt has undergone 28 operations, but he continues to be a fun-loving, well-adjusted little boy. He talks well, and plays with other children at his preschool.

His father discussed Matt's most unusual surgery when he was four. Part of his colon was removed, and used to replace his esophagus which had been removed 15 months before. At the same time, part of his intestine was added to his stomach to enlarge it.

Matt amazed everyone by having a smooth recovery. He's now able to eat food.

Matt's parents are thanking and praising God, as well as giving lots of support to other parents. His father expressed his feelings with a sense of awe toward God's faithfulness. "God has shown us that he's still with us by the wonderful recovery Matt had from these two major operations. He's had no complications. We kept believing that God would eventually come through—and he really has."

PRAYERS

Facing Bad News

Lord, just when we thought things were getting better, the doctor came with bad news. He's plunged into more lab tests and medical evaluations. Our child's symptoms don't look good at all.

My mind is whirling with "what-ifs." I'm waking up in the middle of the night, and I'm nervous during the day. Our friends seem far away—in another world.

Dear God, it's dangerous to jump ahead in anxious thoughts, and I know it. So I come to you. Help me to rest beside your still waters for at least a little while. I give you these fears of the unknown. I thank you that I'm learning to pray, and to release things to you. Why didn't I do it sooner?

Your presence is very real to me, and I sense a new firmness in faith within me—no matter what. Thank you, Lord, for touching this situation right now.

"He will have no fear of bad news; his heart is steadfast, trusting in the Lord" (Ps. 112:7).

"I sought the Lord, and he answered me; he delivered me from all my fears" (Ps. 34:4).

A Lift from Pastoral Care

Lord, thank you especially for your shepherds who often come to our side at just the right time. May we be mature enough to be not disappointed when they can't come. Thank you for our pastor, an instrument of your love and wisdom. He has gently touched the hurting place of our hearts through listening, and praying, and applying the healing balm of the Scriptures. Such ministry is not a short-lived pacifier, but a demonstration of your continuous power!

We are grateful, too, for the hospital chaplain who treats us as though we were the only family on the floor. When I was greatly distressed and felt abandoned, he told me: "Down through the ages many believers have come to a point of feeling forsaken by God. It happens to most of us sometime—as it is for you now. Even Jesus, who was totally obedient in going to the cross, cried out, 'My God, my God, why hast thou forsaken me?' "

I've pondered those thoughts: You *didn't* forsake Jesus in the end, nor will you ever leave us. By sending us pastors, priests and chaplains, you are showing that we are hardly forsaken!

"Then I will give you shepherds after my own heart, who will lead you with knowledge and understanding" (Jer. 3:15).

PART FIVE

I Will Help You

My Help

"I lift up my eyes
to the hills.
From whence does my help come?"

My help comes from our Lord . . .
as I perceive his presence
while climbing with dear ones
those awesome trails
at a child's pace.

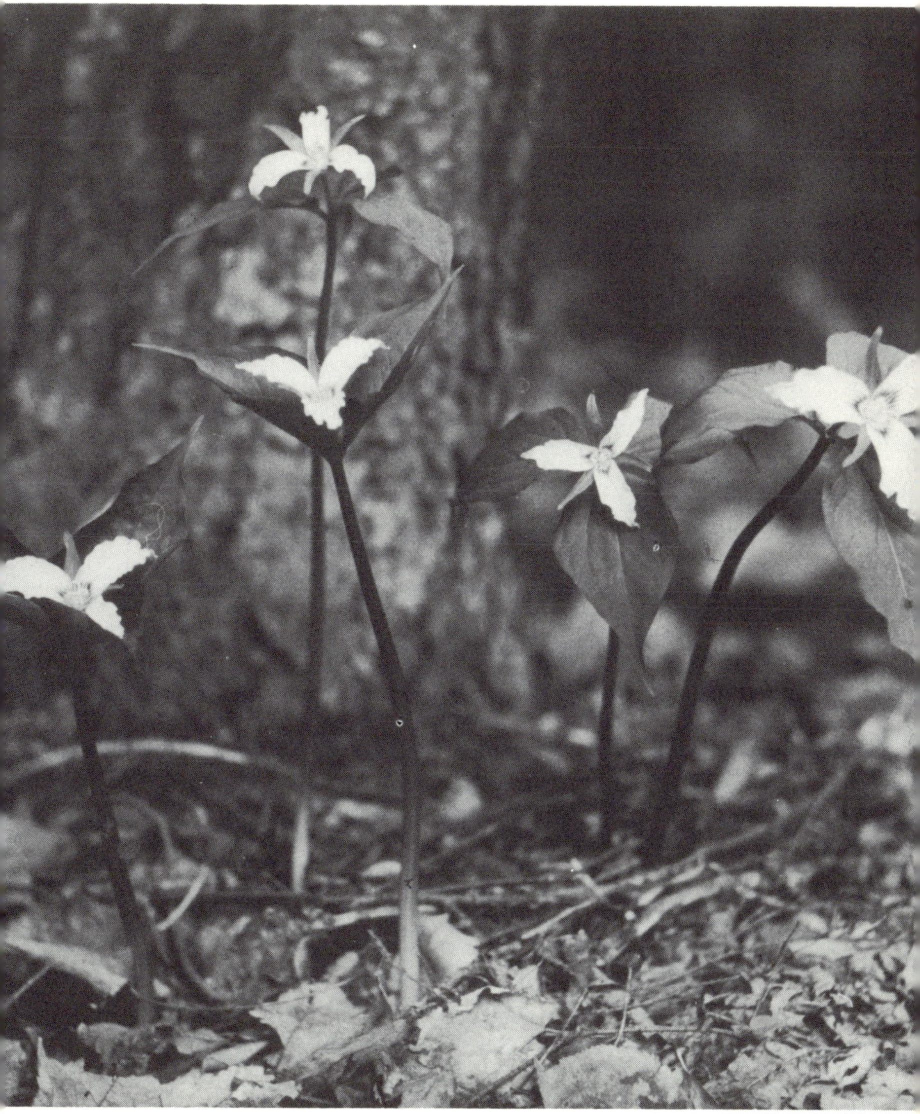

Life Excerpt

Terminal! Treated! Cured!

Eight years ago when Becky was three, she was diagnosed as having a vicious form of cancer which in 95% of similar cases takes a child's life within two years.

After Becky's exploratory surgery, her parents were told she had an inoperable malignant tumor, as well as malignancy in most lymph glands examined. She would be fortunate to live two years.

"It seemed that my world had ended," her father recalls. "The shock was incredible."

Little Becky received 20 days of radiation therapy, then drug therapy. Her parents, Paul and Elizabeth, suffered chronic anxiety and actual mourning. Many times in that first year they worried: Will our child be alive in the morning?

Paul and Elizabeth drew on their Christian faith, prayed together, and asked everyone they knew to pray for Becky. They were upheld especially by Christian friends, clergy, and members of a prayer group they attended regularly. Elizabeth's voice broke as she remembered the prayers of so many who believe in God's power to heal: "We just *besieged* heaven!"

Paul recalls his silent prayer one morning in church: "I *demanded* of the Lord that he heal my daughter. I was a little shocked at my boldness, but the feeling of peace that came sustained me over the months."

About a year after Becky's diagnosis, the doctors scheduled a "second-look operation." In this surgery, one-third of her right adrenal gland, which was the former tumor bed, was removed. The pathology report showed not only zero percent malignancy, but also the presence of normal, healthy ganglion cells.

"The theory of radiation and chemotherapy is not to produce healthy cells," Paul explains, "but to kill malignant cells and even healthy ones simultaneously. Consequently, there's medical evidence that Becky is totally free of malignancy."

Paul and Elizabeth and their family were overjoyed to hear the lab reports, but they were also stunned. "The only thing that the doctors were able to say," reports Elizabeth, "is that they don't know how Becky was cured, and that medical science can't take full credit for it."

"In Becky's case there is no documentation to indicate that an instantaneous cure took place," adds Paul. "It isn't that kind of healing."

Becky's parents believe this now-documented cure was the result of the fervent prayers of a lot of people. They cite medical therapies as another key element God used. Yet Paul and Elizabeth couldn't help asking, "Why us? Why our daughter—when there are so many others needing healing?" They still have no answers. Nor do they have a winning formula as to what brings deliverance from serious illness. Why some are healed and others are not continues to be an age-old mystery.

How did these parents react to the healing of their daughter? "Here you touch a subject that almost nobody has talked about," Elizabeth stresses, "that is, the difficulty of accepting a healing. We human beings don't seem to be as programmed to expect happiness as we are steeled against misfortune."

After her daughter's wonderful medical reports, Elizabeth was utterly relieved, yet physically exhausted. As months went by her strength returned. "We have met others besides ourselves," she explains, "who have found it difficult to deal with a healing—fearful of what the Lord wanted in return, fearful of how to live up to it. There are all kinds of artificial expectations we put on ourselves."

Paul and Elizabeth now see God's blessings of any kind as part of his *unconditional* love. In time they were able to shift gears freely into much praise and thanksgiving to God. A special service of thanks for Becky's healing was even held in their church.

Becky and her parents have grown immensely in their relationship to God. "Praying with Becky and for her healing," reflects Paul, "created a consciousness of the presence of the Lord that I had not known before." And he advises other parents of seriously ill children: "Hope in the Lord. Pray. You're not going to change the mind of God, but you'll change your own heart—to love better and to be a better Christian. And expect a miracle, because miracles happen all the time."

Becky's mother reports that Becky remains healthy, and plays basketball on her grade school team. She is very active in scouting and plays the piano. She enjoyed swimming and horseback riding at Girl Scout camp. She continues to return to the hospital annually for check-ups. And her family continues to praise God.

Even today Becky's cure is a medical puzzle. Parents are seeing more and more marvelous medical puzzles—long remissions, unusual health improvements, complete cures. "In my terms," says Paul, "it's a sign that the Lord is alive and acting in our time." Others call it the alleluia on the victory side of pain.

"When he heard this, Jesus said, 'This sickness will not end in death. No, it is for God's glory so that God's Son may be glorified through it'" (John 11:4).

"Now to him who is able to do immeasurably more than all we ask or imagine, according to his power that is at work within us, to him be glory in the church and in Christ Jesus throughout all generations, for ever and ever! Amen" (Eph. 3:20-21).

PRAYERS

Our Child Is Well!

Almighty and merciful God, our hearts sing today to know that a rough battle has been won! The doctor says our child has fully recovered, and will need no more medical treatment. We thank you; we thank you! We love you.

We look back over the hours in doctors' waiting rooms, and the days of confusion, upset and suffering. But you entered into it all. You were there minute by minute—even though, at times, we forgot you.

Like one of the lepers whom Jesus healed in his day, we come running back; this time with our healthy child, praising you! We are literally dancing around our house.

At this time of celebrating and enjoying the smiles on our child's face, we realize that you have equipped us through this experience. We will have more time these days to serve you in joy, in sensitivity to the needs of others, and in new compassion. Show us ways we can help others through your magnificent love. Help us all to continue in the spirit of thanksgiving we have today. O powerful Lord, we want to truly glorify you forever and ever!

"You will stand firm and without fear. You will surely forget your trouble, recalling it only as waters gone by. Life will be brighter than noonday, and darkness will become like morning" (Job 11:15-17).

My Lord and Savior

Your love, Jesus, has found me over and over again. But it has taken me a long time to really meet you as Jesus the Christ. And how my heart sings!

I'm truly ashamed of all my separation from you. That's sin. Please forgive me for all that sinfulness clothed in self-centeredness. I lived as though I were the center of the universe! I choose now to exalt you as the center, and to dwell in you—and you in me.

Your ministry as the Son of God on earth overflowed with unconditional love for people just like me. You gave your all in sacrificial death on the cross. You rose from the dead through the mighty power of God's eternal plan for mankind. Thank you, dear Master, for sending the Comforter, the Holy Spirit, who drew me to you.

You told us, "The kingdom of heaven is within you." What blessings that brings as I face the trials of life! And what wonder to know that you have promised eternal life to sinners like me who receive you as Lord and Savior. I'm eager to share my decision in the company of others. More than anything I yearn to grow as a newborn creature in you, Jesus, and to follow you, and to serve you, in love and joy every day! Praise your name!

"And this is the testimony: God has given us eternal life, and this is life in his Son. He who has the Son has life; he who does not have the Son of God does not have life" (1 John 5:11-12).

"Yet to all who received him, to those who believed in his name, he gave the right to become children of God" (John 1:12).

Do Not Fear

Do not fear
what may happen tomorrow
The same loving Father
who cares for you today
will care for you tomorrow
and every day.
Either he will shield you
from suffering
or he will give you
unfailing strength
to bear it.
Be at peace, then,
and put aside all
anxious thoughts
and imaginings.

—*St. Francis de Sales*

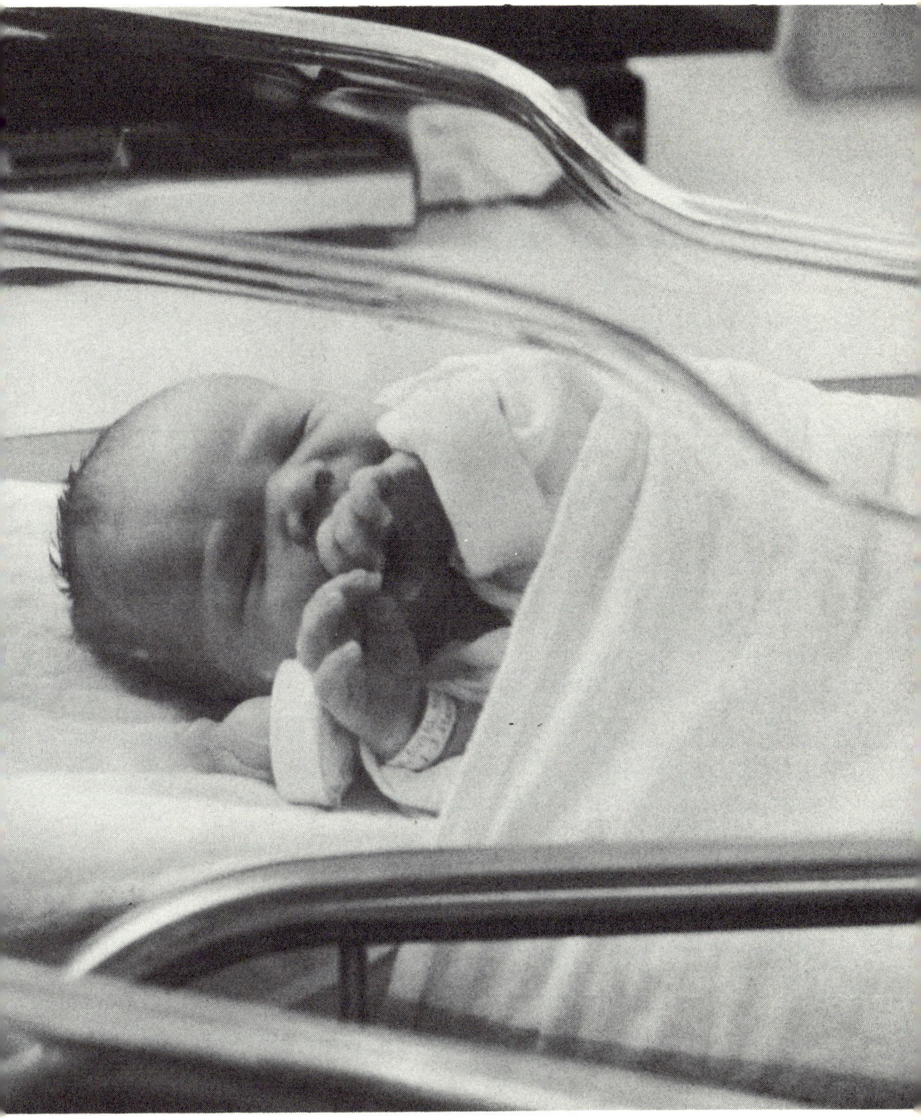

LIFE EXCERPT

What Would You Tell Other Parents?

Parents undergoing the stinging experience of caring for a sick or injured child often express the kinship they feel with others in similar situations. When I met with a variety of parents, I often asked, "What would you like to share with others?" Here are a few of the responses.

• Doris' 11-year-old son Bobby has bone cancer. He has undergone a leg amputation and much chemotherapy. Doris says, "After a child's treatment is underway, it becomes more than a medical problem, but an emotional one for the whole family. There's where the battle is. In our case, our marriage has become stronger through our experience with Bobby's illness. We've held each other up. For some couples, the relationship falls apart. You must keep working at your marriage."

She advises other parents: "When your child is functioning well and is not in the hospital, choose not to consider him sick. Treat him in every way possible as a normal child—discipline and all!"

• Ron, whose son fought leukemia, says, "We were told not to be bitter about the disease that came to our child, but to be grateful to God for the time he gave us with him. That isn't easy, but I've come to the deep sense that our child essentially belongs to God."

• Margaret, the mother of a handicapped child, stresses, "You may feel as though you are the only person in the world who feels a certain way. Find someone to confide in. You can't do it alone."

• "God does let us hit low places so that we can work through our need and come into dependence on him," says Nancy. "When I let him take the lead through the Holy Spirit, I find I'm more effective in dealing with my teenaged daughter who suffers from the complexities of *anorexia nervosa*."

• "Our baby daughter went through many critical episodes because of a heart defect," Janice relates. "One time when she was in ICU, I prayed, 'God, this is *all* I can take!' I thought I was going to snap mentally from the strain. Within hours she was stable enough to go into successful heart surgery. I'm convinced that God hears our prayers."

• The mother of a younger child adds, "The sweetest times I've had with my child is when we've prayed together for other sick children. It does something for us both. Perhaps we're experiencing the healing side effects of prayer. I think of Job in the Bible who was restored *after* he prayed for his friends.

• Judy, whose child has terminal cancer, says candidly: "I discovered that self-centeredness is a trap—even if your child is dying. One time as I sat in church, I thought, 'Oh, if people only knew what I'm going through!' It was during times of self-centeredness and self-pity that I was thrown off balance emotionally. I sank into depression. Since then I've learned that the only healthful pattern is to center on God, on others, and on your child. When I do that, I'm much more effective as a mother to a child who desperately needs me."

• "We had a baby with serious birth defects who fought constantly for his life," Kay recalls. "Many times we had the feeling of putting him in Jesus' arms in utter trust. But even when you live by faith, there is a reservoir of grief that stays with you—a deep lingering hurt for your child. So I tell other parents: God and medical science might still come through with a cure for your child. Keep up hope!"

LIFE EXCERPT

A Father's Signal at Night

As I interviewed parents, one of my own experiences as a mother came vividly to memory.

"I hate to see you leave," I said to my husband as he started to turn from our baby's hospital bed. Our 18-month-old son, wiggling in an oxygen tent, was finally winning over a bout with a respiratory infection.

Bob smiled good-bye to our son, then kissed me gently. "Visiting hours are over; I really have to go," he said, just as I spotted a firm-faced nurse filling the doorway.

"Look down there," he added, pointing through the window to where the car was parked. "I'll be driving right past your room. Stand here at the window. When I come by I'll blink my lights. It'll be my little signal that I love you two, and I'll be thinking of you."

Minutes later I recognized our car as it slowly moved on the street below. The lights blinked on, then off. A few more feet and another blink, and then another. As it turned onto the main street, another. The lights kept blinking until my blurred eyes could no longer see them. Then I noticed the stars of God's heavens. They were blinking too—*I love you. I love you.* And I thought, Isn't that the signal God wants for all of his children every night?

"Every good and perfect gift is from above, coming down from the Father of the heavenly lights, who does not change like shifting shadows" (James 1:17).

PRAYERS

Time for Me

Heavenly Father, I thank you for leading me to think of my own needs today; to take a day off. What a tonic it was to have lunch with a friend, and to slip aside my preoccupation with our child's health.

It was refreshing to munch potato chips and talk of good books we've read and places we've been. My tight muscles relaxed as my friend stirred me to a hearty laugh.

I felt stronger when I was able to say to my companion, "Let's not focus on any problems today. Let's just enjoy our time together." It worked. I felt joy soar within me as I looked into the face of a wonderful friend. I savor the satisfactions of this friendship—and we've even planned a morning on the tennis court.

Thank you, God, thank you! I feel so new again.

"Taste and see that the Lord is good" (Ps. 34:8).

"Pleasant words are a honeycomb, sweet to the soul and healing to the bones" (Prov. 16:24).

Our Marriage

Heavenly Father, we thank you for allowing us to enter into a wonderful union, and for us to become parents. I thank you for the great blessings through the special one I married.

I'm very concerned these days, for our marriage is under a subtle strain. The demands of our child needing constant care seem to be driving us apart. We rush past each other. We are so absorbed in our children that our private moments seem to dissolve.

I'm thankful that we've become aware of our tendency to slip away from each other. May this be an opportunity for sensitivity to each other's needs and for growth.

Come, Lord, into the center of our marriage. We belong to each other and to you. You can help us back into balance, even amid crises. Show us once again how to be best friends as well as loving mates. We want renewed sweetness and creativity in our life together. Help us to discover ways to guard our privacy, and grant us moments to look into each other's eyes with that deep, believing love.

We've heard that a child's long-term illness can jar a couple's relationship *or* draw them in powerful closeness. We want to walk and to talk together in the rhythm of oneness and victorious love! Hear these, our hearts' desires, Father, and bless our marriage.

"Haven't you read . . . that at the beginning the Creator 'made them male and female,' and said, 'For this reason a man will leave his father and mother and be united to his wife, and the two will become one flesh'?" (Matt. 19:4-5).

Part Six

I Will Uphold You with My Victorious Right Hand

In the Pocket of My Soul

I have a prayer . . .
a prayer in the pocket of my soul.
I turn that pocket
inside-out before you.
Do your work now, Lord.
Slip a living song down deep
into the pocket of my soul.
A song of victory.

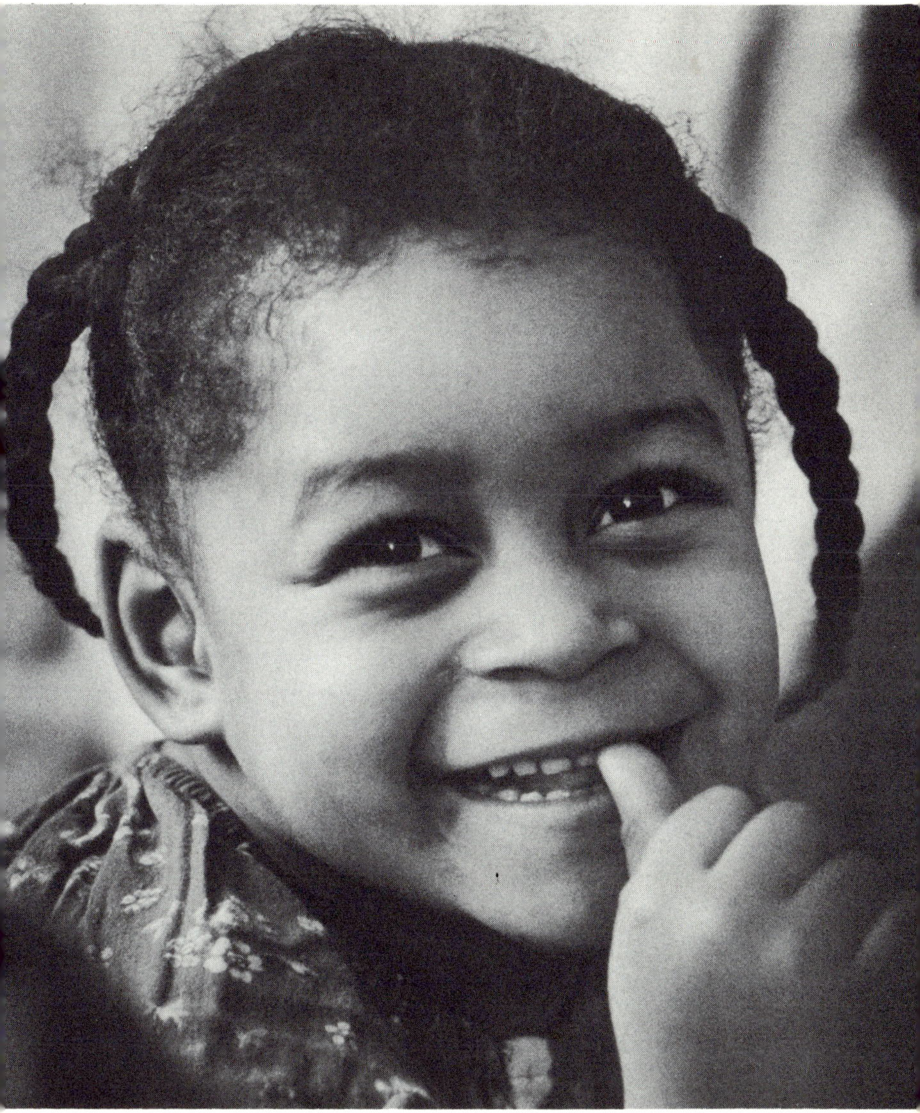

LIFE EXCERPT

Beacons from the Life of a Teenager

Mark Heil and his younger sister, Diana, used to jump on the bed, trampoline-style, giggling and singing at the top of their voices. Moments when their parents were absent set the stage for such great, silly fun.

Mark leaped at chances to have a good time during long periods of remission from leukemia. He fought the disease valiantly since its onset when he was six and a half. Whenever possible he poured himself into many vigorous endeavors. He loved to fish, water ski, ice skate, and play tennis with his dad. He was good at all of them. And even leukemia didn't stop this handsome, big-boned blond from eager quality living.

" 'For in him we live and move and have our being' is a verse that really described Mark's way of life," comments his mother Alberta. "He chose to live in Christ. He experienced the abundant life, the exuberant life, the life of faith, joy, and love. He also had the power in his life to fight the little trials as well as the *big* one he was enduring."

Seven years of battle with a life-threatening disease brought all kinds of trials for Mark, such as long hours as an outpatient at the hospital. There he endured many vein injections, lumbar punctures and bone marrow procedures. He suffered some severe headaches when the disease infiltrated his central nervous system. Yet Mark, unknowingly, showed others how to endure pain, uncertainty, and physical weakness, as he continued to face the day-to-day challenges of junior high. He started eighth grade having gained weight and wearing a wig for the first time, both the result of chemotherapy. He came home and told his family, "The kids say I look different." Yet he shook off self-consciousness with a previously made decision: "I've decided that no matter what happens, I'm going to be me."

"Mark went on and lived," recalls his mother, "not looking at the circumstances very much. He enjoyed life and loved people. He was always ready to laugh. Once he commented, 'When I feel down, I just eat some chicken noodle soup!' He insisted it lifted his spirits."

Because of periods of absence, Mark fell behind in schoolwork. Yet he appreciated the rigors of studying. Alberta remembers Mark once pushing to catch up on homework all in one evening. He came in that night, flopped on the couch, and said, "Boy, it feels good to work hard!"

A few months before Mark died, he was interviewed on the radio by his pastor. Mark told the listening audience, "Jesus really came into my life about a year ago. I've known about Jesus ever since I was a little kid, but I finally accepted him as my Lord and Savior. We can't live without him and be happy."

He went on to explain, "At church I've met a lot of new friends, and I think I've helped them in some things I've learned in Christ—and they've really helped *me*." During the broadcast Mark never referred to his illness. He was very private about it, not even discussing it with friends. He wanted to live above his condition, and to be treated as a "regular guy." He shunned pity.

Mark's father Ron was especially close, not only as a dad, but as a friend. Ron says, "I was constantly thankful to see Mark living in God's grace and power. It was a strength to us all."

Mark had a way of making others feel very special when he talked with them. Toward the end of his life when his strength was slipping away, he remained sensitive to the needs of those he loved. One day he saw his mother immersed in her Bible. Her face must have revealed her heavy heart. "*Don't worry*, Mom," he said lovingly. "That's what God's for."

Diana noted his calmness and lack of fear throughout the roughest days. Even now one of her favorite Scripture songs is: "The Lord is my light and my salvation—whom shall I fear? The Lord is the stronghold of my life—of whom shall I be afraid?" (Ps. 27:1).

Ron observed that Mark went beyond positive thinking in dealing with suffering. "Mark believed God's Word and loved it," he says. "He was truly fed by it." His parents read the Bible to him every night, or he read to them.

About two weeks before Mark died, he told his pastor again that he had given his life completely to Christ. "Jesus can do whatever he wants to with my life," Mark declared. "He can take me now, if he wants to." Mark surrendered his life, while maintaining a spirit that never gave up.

Mark's life was unique, and demonstrated an amazing capacity to adjust to great odds. He lived fully in his rich relationships with the Lord, his family and his friends. Many still remember his courage and poise as a young person with a winning smile, even during the traumas of medical battle. But I think he would say that these attributes were by-products of his fellowship with the Lord. In almost 14 years with us, Mark Heil spread lavish and unforgettable blessings for many people. Truly he taught us.

"Thou dost keep him in perfect peace, whose mind is stayed on thee, because he trusts in thee" (Isa. 26:3 RSV).

Prayers

Courage Contagious

Lord God, I think over the uncertainties of life our family has already experienced. As darkness and pain spread upon us, I've seen you illuminate the moment. I've witnessed a flow of indescribable power through the compassion and skill of doctors, nurses, and chaplains. I've viewed it gratefully in a Christian friend's love-filled eyes. Most of all, I've seen it as our child took conquering steps up a jagged mountain of physical disability. I call all this courage contagious.

I search for the source of such ruggedness amid a drawn-out medical battle. It must be of your Holy Spirit, touching a person in need, who in turn touches others. I see now how courage has enveloped our family during this time of strain. I praise you and thank you for your work!

As I ponder your power, I remember Jesus in his acute redemptive suffering on a cross when he looked after his agonizing neighbor who hung beside him. I know now that Jesus Christ supplies us with all strength, all love, all wisdom—and all courage. His Spirit is truly contagious.

"Jesus Christ is the same yesterday and today and forever" (Heb. 13:8).

"I can do everything through him who gives me strength" (Phil. 4:13).

LIFE EXCERPT

Toward the End of a Journey

Nothing could have kept me from going to be with my twin sister and her family that Friday afternoon in early April 1976. Still, as my bus sped across Missouri, I felt stirrings of apprehension. Mark's medical reports continued to show he was sliding rapidly downhill. Remission had eluded him for many months. Now the disease was out of control. How would Mark be? How would his family be coping?

When Alberta met my bus, that special love and closeness we know as twins bounded into full force. I immediately knew when I saw her: the burden was heavy. We hugged. As soon as we got to the car, she began to cry softly, and I wrapped my arms around her.

"Mark had a check-up today," she said. "After the doctor saw the reports, he talked with me alone—and he called Ron. There is nothing more medical science can do." Her voice broke. "He said Mark could die anytime—even in the next three days."

I was stunned.

As we drove to the house, Alberta shared her reaction to the heartbreaking news. She and Ron trusted God and viewed the doctors as a means through which God works. But they were in no way giving up hope.

Mark was resting in bed, watching TV with his sister Diana. When he saw me, a broad smile danced across the pallor of his face. We chatted. Oh, the sweetness of his spirit! And such a calm maturity for a boy about to turn 14.

Alberta told me that, although Mark had not been told the grim news, he knew he needed a miracle. That morning his pain had become suddenly fierce, and he had prayed with her for a miracle.

Alberta, Ron, and Diana moved with amazing naturalness that evening. One might have expected emotional chaos to spring up at any point. But it didn't. Instead, I saw a serenity in Ron and Alberta—a steadfastness. They talked with me, sharing their grief. Yet there was no panic; no self-pity. They were living one moment at a time.

Beautiful love for one another was the hallmark of their home. And we all savored just being with Mark. That night I started a sketchy journal about my visit. I wrote, "The peace and presence of God is very real in this house. What a comfort!"

What were the ingredients for such a climate at this time of crisis? Alberta had written me:

> I'm keeping a brief diary of Mark's happy experiences, a record of God's blessings. It has helped

> me to focus on the good, the lovely, and whatever is worthy of praise. I take time to just notice and enjoy Mark, and I count each day as a gift from God for him—and us.
>
> Each one of us has come to know the love and power of the Lord in a deeper way. But we have hardly "arrived" in our growth. Jesus has arrived on the scene. We invited him a long time ago. We *must* keep looking to him.

Ron and Alberta had prayed earnestly for permanent remission, for protection from infection and serious treatment side effects, including the loss of his hair. So many of these prayers were answered! Mark stayed in bone marrow remission for five years. He skipped many expected infections. Remarkably, he kept his thick blond hair through his first six years of chemotherapy. And in seven years, he spent only four days in the hospital.

Yet there were times of disappointment. "I remember one time Mark and I prayed together in frustration about his condition," Ron recalls. "We asked, 'God, *what* are you doing?' "

Now, during my visit, *I* was wondering what God was doing. The morning after my arrival, there was a noticeable change in Mark. He was rallying! His pain was under control. I saw him eat pancakes, walk around, and we played a game at the table.

"Mark, you're having a good day," I commented.

"You revived me," he returned with a warm smile. I was touched, but I knew God was answering all the prayers being offered every day for him.

Each day, miraculously, Mark gained strength. One night his grandparents took us all out to dinner. Mark moved slowly, but he was able to partake and enjoy. He further amazed us by going to church and Sunday school the next day. God, in his faithfulness, was upholding not only Mark, but all of us.

Alberta and Ron's journey with Mark had many of the painful elements that thousands of other parents go through. There was the anguish and inner grieving when Mark had a relapse; exhausting days when he needed special care; and many trips to the hospital. They worked through cycles of anxiety, heartache and sleepless nights. But as I viewed them in April 1976, I could see what conquerors they had become! Cycles of uncontrolled fear no longer had power over them.

"It's the day-to-day walk with the Lord that really makes a difference," Ron says. "If you have a good relationship with God through Christ, he will work on problems like fear and bitterness through grace. The key is coming to a place where you *trust the Lord.*" Like many parents, they had grown in their capacity for crisis.

Ron also stressed a practical approach. "I tried to go on with life much the same as I always had," he says of those days. "We did not try to compensate for Mark's illness by giving him things." Instead, he and Alberta offered meaningful and fun experiences. They majored in good relationships, not only with the Lord, but with other people. It was a love priority. Then, when the floods came in Mark's condition that April, their house was built upon a rock—and they stood upright and equipped for whatever might come.

On the last morning of my visit, Mark got ready to go to school for a few hours—another miracle! Ron asked the four of us to gather with him in a prayer circle to thank God for my visit. I was holding Mark's hand, and praying silently I wouldn't break into tears. My throat tightened as we kissed good-bye. "I love you, Mark," I whispered.

He climbed into the car with his father. I stood on the porch, a forced smile quivering on my face. I waved. I waved again. I knew they couldn't hear me weep as they drove slowly away. Mark sat so tall and straight, so pale. The car turned so I could no longer see them. "O dear God," I prayed, "hold him close—no matter what happens—hold him close!" I was surely echoing the prayers of all who loved him.

Looking back on those last days with Mark, Alberta now comments on the vital helps that got her through:

"My husband's support was tremendous. We talked out everything, we prayed together, we were active in Christian groups. Several close friends were my outlets for sharing, and for prayer requests. Two of those friends were my mother and father."

Ron and Alberta had many times of intimate sharing with their pastor. When Mark slipped out of remission, he asked them, "Have you surrendered Mark to God?"

"We answered an honest yes," Alberta remembers, "even though we were still praying earnestly for healing. And we never forgot what our pastor had told

Mark: *There is nothing about death to be afraid of for a Christian.*"

Mark's journey drew to a close during Holy Week, 1976—two weeks after my visit. On Maundy Thursday evening he received his last solid food, Holy Communion, lovingly brought by elders of the church. On Good Friday morning, his nose began to bleed. It wouldn't stop.

Alberta shares glimpses of the experience:

Friday, April 16—The copious nosebleed continued all Good Friday. By nightfall the doctor sent Mark to the hospital, giving a "stat" order for blood platelets. Ron tenderly carried him to the car. As we drove the familiar route, Mark broke the silence. "I forgot my wig—but it doesn't matter."

The blood platelet transfusion was administered to Mark; no medication was given. He was hemorrhaging internally, but suffering no pain. I could feel it—the doctors considered this the end. I was weeping inside.

Our pastor came quickly, and we took turns working with the nosebleed. Mark's doctor came and packed his nose; then gave him a long hug.

He's hugging him good-bye—I thought. I blinked away tears. Then a deep assurance welled up inside of me: *God was in control of Mark's life.* I felt no fear; he was upholding us.

1:00 A.M.: Before our pastor left, we all held hands with Mark and prayed. An indescribable love, sweetness, peace filled the room. Oneness with our Lord—

and with our dear son. Ron slipped his arm around me—more oneness.

Ron and I were numb as we kept the all-night vigil with Mark. We gave him drinks, held his hand, expressed our love.

"Mark, I love everything about you," I said. He smiled. Then dozed a little.

Saturday morning, April 17—Mark's breathing became rapid, but he was alert, and able to drink soda. "Something good has *got* to come out of this," he said.

"Yes, Mark," I replied, "God works all things together for good." He began to breathe faster. I was praying in the depths of my being, crying, "Help!" to God—"Help Mark."

Ron kept his hand on Mark's shoulder. "God is with you, Mark," he repeated over and over in his strong, loving tone. Our pastor slipped into the room.

Silence. Utter stillness—except for Mark's labored breathing.

Mark gazed past all of us, looking straight ahead: *"I see Jesus!"*

Instantly we began hugging him, all of us thanking God at once. Victory was in the air, but I wasn't sure what was happening. Mark's eyes were shining. Tears were streaming down my face. I cried, "Thank you, Lord, thank you!"

Within 30 minutes our son died. In distant parts of the world, Easter morning was already breaking forth with all Christ's promises of eternal life. Mark was personally receiving the fulfillment of those promises—to live "ever with the Lord."

Prayer

When Death Comes

Father in heaven, this is my most personal prayer of all. Our child is gone—*much too soon*. Oh, how I miss this one I love so deeply! In silence my innermost being cries to you. . . . Thoughts and memories whirl in my mind—beautiful memories that will never die.

I must take time to pour out my feelings, to grieve, and to let go. To survive I must surrender all of these painful puzzles of life into your hands. Please help me.

Every parent's prayer is so different. For me, the hush of your presence sustains me. *Thank you* for our child's days with us—our wonderful child. I praise you for the assurance of eternal life through Christ, and the trust that our child dwells with you forever.

I think of what one mother said about seeing her son die. "Spiritually, it is a peaceful, spectacular event—the moment of death." I want to believe that. I thank you that our child did not go alone to heaven. You are enfolding our dear one with your everlasting love right now—please include my love!

Even in this aching loss, I believe you have a plan of victory for us all. Lead us gently forward, Lord, to live in that victory to your glory.

" 'For my thoughts are not your thoughts, neither are your ways my ways' declares the Lord. 'As the heavens are higher than the earth, so are my

ways higher than your ways and my thoughts than your thoughts'" (Isa. 55:8-9).

A Winding Path

Dead End, I thought—
with so much pain
and darkness.
But God marked it
Detour
with a steady light
on his larger plan,
revealed over months
of following him.

CENTRAL UNITED METHODIST
CHILDREN'S LIBRARY